Focus on Solutions
A Health Professional's Guide

Focus on Solutions
A Health Professional's Guide

KIDGE BURNS BA, PGDipSLT
Chelsea and Westminster Hospital, London

W
WHURR PUBLISHERS
LONDON AND PHILADELPHIA

First Published 2005
Whurr Publishers Ltd
19b Compton Terrace, London N1 2UN, England and
325 Chestnut Street, Philadelphia PA 19106, USA

Reprinted 2005

British Library Cataloguing in Publication Data

A catalogue record for this book is available from the
British Library.

ISBN 186156 479 1

Printed and bound in the UK by Athenaeum Press Limited,
Gateshead, Tyne & Wear.

Contents

Acknowledgements

Both Steve de Shazer and Insoo Kim Berg are an inspiration on video or in person when they demonstrate their skills with different clients. 'Interviewing for solutions' (De Jong and Berg, 2002) has been extremely helpful for an in-depth description of SFBT.

I am grateful to Harvey Ratner for his comments on Chapter 1. He first helped me to become focused on solutions in 1998 at BRIEF (formerly Brief Therapy Practice) and I have been fortunate to have had training and advice from Harvey since that time. My thanks to the participants on the Solution Focused Therapy listserv (SFT-L) for their lively debates. They have discussed a number of issues raised in this book and have helped me understand how SFBT works within different professions.

The enthusiasm of Stephanie Martin at Whurr to explore the world of SFBT persuaded me to embark on this project and her patience and eye for detail over the past year have been invaluable. In the SLT department at Chelsea and Westminster Hospital my wonderful colleagues Amanda Mozely, Judy Legge and Merida Donald have been most generous in sharing ideas and case examples. Thanks also to Kate Malcomess, Rob Spence, Julia Binder, Pat Lavelle, Didi Prichard and a number of students over the years who have asked useful questions.

I am truly indebted to the many clients who we have been privileged to work with and from whom we have learnt so much. Names and identifying information have been changed to protect client confidentiality but some of them will recognise their own particular humour, courage and insight.

Finally, this book could not have been written without the support of my husband Jimmy and daughters Julia and Miriam, who are a constant source of warmth and love.

Preface

Anyone who is unwell at home or in hospital knows how important it is to be able to look at life beyond 'the problem'. This book gives an account of clients who have been able to find hopes and goals for the future despite struggling with a variety of physical, functional and psychological difficulties. Their quality of life has been helped by a solution focused approach which encourages clients to explore what they want different in their lives.

In 1997 I had been working for four years in North London with an 'elderly' client group (65+). I heard a colleague give a short presentation on Solution Focused Brief Therapy (SFBT) and instantly I was hooked! It sounded as if there was a way of working that treated clients in a more respectful way and that made more sense, especially with an older client group, than much of what I had learnt as a speech and language therapist (SLT) in college.

My enthusiasm for the approach remains as strong today as on that first day, not just because I have learnt more about it through attending training courses, workshops, conferences and reading books but, more importantly, I can see that it works. Both clients and colleagues comment on how SFBT has changed their lives for the better.

This book is a description of how a group of practitioners have used working with solutions to improve their quality of care. I now work in Central London in an acute hospital seeing clients aged 18+ who have either been admitted as inpatients or are seen in the Speech and Language Therapy Department as outpatients. Occasionally I see people in their homes if they become too unwell to come to the hospital. Most of the case examples given in this book are of clients I have seen who have communication and/or swallowing difficulties as a result of a stroke, a stammer, Parkinson's disease, traumatic brain injury, HIV, cancer, voice or memory problems. Unlike many therapy books the chapters here are not divided according to different impairments, since I start from the assumption held by solution focused practitioners that these clients, like anyone else, have common dreams and hopes.

SFBT has become increasingly important in the health and education services. Doctors, psychologists, adult psychiatry teams, health visitors, counsellors and teachers are just some of the professions who have been trained in this approach, and it has also been used in coaching, appraisal and strategic planning in business. There is extensive literature dealing with alcohol and drug abuse, family breakdown or psychiatric problems and how clients have benefited from SFBT. To date, however, there has not been much written on its application with the client group in this book, and whenever I have given any talks on the subject there has always been a keen interest in specific examples. It is for this reason that I agreed to bring together over seventy case examples so that others can read, enjoy and learn from these clients' stories.

It is hoped that whatever your profession — therapist, nurse, doctor or psychologist — you may find something new and of interest. For example, you may not have thought it possible to see a client with significant physical impairment and be persuaded that together you have achieved what they need in only one session.

An introductory chapter to SFBT is given for those who are unfamiliar with what Steve de Shazer would describe as a way of talking rather than an approach. The book is designed to be read from the beginning; when you get to Chapters 4 and 5 you will be familiar with many of the questions included in the sessions described. It aims to address a number of issues that arise from using a different mindset. This challenges some of the ideas held in traditional caseload management and how we involve other professions, students and families in our work. To help demonstrate effectiveness, care aims and outcomes from case examples are included as well as data from studies that have used SFBT.

Chapter 1
Introduction to Solution Focused Brief Therapy

Traditionally, scientists have measured the outcomes of health conditions by relying on mortality data. More recently, the international concern about health care outcomes has shifted to the assessment of functioning at the level of the whole human being, in day-to-day life. (WHO, 2002)

Since the first version of the International Classification of Functioning, Disability and Health (ICF), which provides a language and framework for the description of health and disability, was published in 1980 there has been a shift in emphasis from looking at people's disabilities to focusing on their level of health. There is now the recognition that it can be more helpful to measure the impact rather than the level of impairment itself.

Disability is an interaction between features within a person and the context within which they live, so that both medical and social responses are appropriate. Some aspects of disability however are 'entirely internal to the person, while another aspect is almost entirely external' (WHO, 2002). To reflect the biological, individual and social aspects of health, the ICF disability and functioning are viewed as interactions between health conditions and contextual factors. They consider body structure and function, activity and participation (the whole person and how they function in a social context) and environmental/attitudinal factors.

There is growing awareness of the importance of psychosocial elements in health care. Crises can undermine clients' self-esteem and belief in their own personal competence, and while clinicians spend a considerable amount of time analysing the output and input abilities of clients with communication difficulties, less time is given to looking at the levels of depression or anxiety of clients or their carers (Brumfitt, 1998). You may feel such areas require lengthy, in-depth help beyond your level of expertise. But effective rehabilitation needs the environmental and attitudinal areas addressed, and a psychologist, social worker or counsellor may not be readily available.

Solution Focused Brief Therapy (SFBT) can generate a feeling of hope towards achieving change and it has the ability to promote a more positive attitude towards problems or disabilities. The approach assists clients and carers in realizing that they are capable of getting through a crisis. It gives anyone working within the hospital, school or home environment a set of tools to work with so that clients can deal with emotional issues more effectively as well as establish goals more easily for day-to-day functioning. There is a simplicity about it which is often lacking in other models of therapy, and because it translates what the client is feeling into very practical 'doing' activities, it fits well into our case management.

SFBT helps you assume competency in yourself and in those with whom you work. It encourages change to be seen in small steps, rather than the team thinking in absolutes where results are seen as good or bad.

History of solution focus

'Solution Focused Brief Therapy' was pioneered through the work of Steve de Shazer, Insoo Kim Berg and their colleagues at the Brief Family Therapy Center (BFTC) in Milwaukee, Wisconsin (brief-therapy.org), the term first being coined in 1982. Drawing on the tradition of family therapy and the work of Milton Erickson (Cade and O'Hanlon, 1993) the approach has evolved over time, and includes a number of theoretical approaches; cognitive, behavioural, narrative, experiential and systemic. Working with individuals, couples and families to resolve a wide variety of difficulties, they have trained many professionals in their procedures at the BFTC and around the world.

> Whatever the cause of a problem might be, its continuation has something to do with the context or setting in which it occurs and the expectation that the problem is going to continue ... This assumption leads to the idea that any difference in behaviour, thoughts, feelings, perceptions, and/or context stands a chance of making a difference such that the complaint is resolved. (de Shazer, 1988, p. 57)

Exploring problem behaviour, de Shazer noticed there are times when the problem appears less or is absent altogether. An example he gives is of a depressed client who is able to describe times when he is slightly less depressed. This is called 'the exception to the rule'. When asked how he manages to do this, the client is able to identify some of his own resources and strengths that he is using to solve the problem. These exceptions form the basis to showing the client possible solutions towards moving forward.

Working on the 'solution' pattern of behaviours de Shazer noticed they begin to outweigh the problem patterns. As he does more of the things that help improve his mood, the client becomes less depressed.

Brief therapy

Typical of the brief/strategic therapist is the avoidance of an elaborate theory of personality or of dysfunction, and a concern with how to intervene as briefly and as economically as possible (Cade and O'Hanlon, 1993). Meeting the demands of managed care was not, however, the idea behind solution focused therapy. As the team at Milwaukee refined their techniques over 25 years the number of sessions decreased, particularly as interest grew in exploring clients' hopes for the future rather than looking at the problems in the present or the past. 'Following the methods will lead to brief treatment without you forcing yourself to do brief therapy' (Berg and Reuss, 1998).

You will find those who make no distinction between the terms Brief Therapy, Solution Focused Therapy or Solution Focused Brief Therapy. This book will refer to the approach as Solution Focused Brief Therapy which is widely accepted as the Milwaukee Model. The Milwaukee team, still led by Steve de Shazer and Insoo Kim Berg, would be keen to emphasize that rather than using SFBT simply as a set of techniques, it is a way of thinking that follows some basic assumptions (Berg, 1991).

Some basic assumptions

If it ain't broke, don't fix it

Traditional hospital treatment emphasizes a medical, disease-oriented model. In contrast to the medical model, a health-oriented approach defines the client as the authority on what needs to change and how that will happen (Miller, Hubble and Duncan, 1996). This belief that the client is the expert in all aspects of their lives challenges the role of the doctor/therapist/teacher as the expert. You may have considerable expertise in dealing with certain situations but that does not necessarily mean you know all the 'right' or 'wrong' ways for the client to move forward. This accounts for some of the failures of treatment plans that tell clients what to do. Similarly, a client may have developed a way of dealing with a problem that could be classified as 'maladaptive'. A particular strategy used by someone who stammers would be an example of this. If it works for the client, don't fix it. Look into the reasons as to how it is helpful and another strategy may, or may not, emerge as useful to them.

If it works, do more of it

Insoo Kim Berg describes a client, referred as 'suicidal', who walks into her office held up by two people:

Insoo: So ... How do you do that?

Client: Do what?

Insoo: Walk! It takes so much energy to move one foot in front of the other. How do you manage to do that?

When the client explains the reasons for her being able to come to therapy Insoo is able to identify strengths in the client and to come to the conclusion that she isn't at a high risk of self-harm. These strengths can be used by the client in other areas of her life to formulate solutions to her problems, so that the session becomes a time for solution talk rather than problem talk (Berg, 2000). As de Shazer discovered, finding out what the client does that can be utilized to build solutions involves eliciting the right kind of talk.

> If you do not ask about exceptions and successes, the client will not tell you. After all, what they are concerned about is the problem which drove them to seeking therapy. (de Shazer, 1988, p. 158)

Your client may be in hospital with very real and pressing difficulties. Eliciting the 'right kind of talk' should not have the perceived effect of trivializing the problems. Hence the belief that SFBT is simple but not easy, and the best way to become familiar with the kind of questions asked is to watch or read about sessions with clients.

If it doesn't work, do something different

You may find this applies to the clients who have been doing some dysarthria exercises for facial weakness and no apparent or perceived change has occurred. Rather than try and try again, do something different. Finding interventions and suggestions that are individualized to fit each client with unique sets of circumstances is the practitioner's job, and your task is to utilize the changes clients create themselves in the most positive way possible. The Buddhist idea that change is inevitable and happening all the time is an important concept in SFBT, and can be helpful to remember when clients appear to have reached a plateau in their care management. In general system theory, the principle that a difference or change in one part of a system will lead to repercussions in other parts of the system is well established.

Take the example of a client with voice difficulties. The relationship between voice, emotion and physical state has long been recognized by those working with voice (Martin and Darnley, 2004). The client may have tried various suggestions regarding voice care, such as avoiding dry atmospheres or alcohol and resting the voice, but it appears to have made little difference. The difference that makes the difference could be looking at self-esteem; changes in this area will have an effect on the various components that make up the vocal process. Lowered eye levels and slumped shoulders, tension in the shoulders, neck and jaw, shallow breathing patterns and a faster breath rate may all be greatly alleviated if there is some consideration given to a client's level of stress. One change to take some of the stress out of their lives can have a ripple effect towards finding solutions to problems with their voice.

Key points to remember

- If it ain't broke, don't fix it
- If it works, do more of it
- If it doesn't work, do something different

The first session

It may not be possible or desirable to follow a format in the first session. Chapters later in the book will look at situations that arise when a client is seen in a hospital bed as opposed to your office or in their home; factors such as the length of the session and the cognitive abilities or awareness of the client will come into play and will determine what you can or can't do. A number of steps, however, can be used as a reference for core first and follow-up session structure. At the Speech and Language Therapy Department in the Chelsea and Westminster Hospital we have found the following headings useful. Based on those given to us when we were trained by BRIEF in London some years ago, we continue to find them useful today with our varied caseload.

Problem-free talk

How you start a session with a client can communicate very clearly how you view the client as a person rather than a problem. A key way to demonstrate this is to engage in what is referred to in SFBT as problem-free talk.

For example, a client who has been referred for a swallowing assessment in hospital would not be asked immediately about difficulties associated with eating and drinking. If a client with Parkinson's disease (PD) comes into your office as an outpatient and shows considerable difficulty getting into a chair, you would acknowledge this ('Take your time', 'It can be tricky, can't it?') but the aim would be to avoid if possible a lengthy discussion on their reduced mobility as a start to the session. The difference between problem-free talk and social chit-chat is that 'the therapist is on the look-out for clients' strengths and resources which may be helpful in resolving the problem'

(Sharry, Madden and Darmody, 2001). Asking the client with PD how the day is outside, or noticing some flowers by a patient's bedside allows you to connect with clients as people and can give immediate insight into their strengths and support systems.

Many would say that they already do this. In SFBT it is not only the practitioners' questions and comments that matter, but how the clients answer that help you focus on the next step. The person with physical difficulties may tell you that it's pouring with rain, the taxi didn't arrive and they got lost getting to your office:

Therapist: So despite the rain, the taxi and getting lost, you arrived here on time! How did you manage that?

Client: I'm very stubborn and determined. And I always allow a lot of time in case something happens.

Therapist: Have you always been such a determined and organized person?

Not only has the client been able to recognize strengths in himself, but the therapist can compliment him and use them to explore other examples of when these existing resources are used by the client to overcome difficulties. And all within a few minutes of the client coming in through the door!

Problem definition

Moving on to what the client hopes to achieve by coming to therapy, you need to establish clear client-centred goals to ensure an effective outcome. Clients need to say in their own words what they want to work on, and it is sometimes surprising how different their perceptions are from those who referred them.

Consider the case of a 61-year-old client with Parkinson's disease who was referred by his doctor for help with his 'huskiness of voice'.

Therapist: Your doctor has referred you here. Perhaps you'd like to tell me in your own words ... How can I be helpful to you?

Client: I have a weak voice as a result of Parkinson's disease. I dribble a bit. Sometimes I have a problem with my swallow. None of them are chronic but they bother me. My consultant gave me the impression that I should just get on with it, but the thing is ... it's happening to me, not to him ... and I would like some help.

Notice the initial question. You don't ask 'What's the problem with your voice?' You ask an open ended question, which in this example allows the client to list clearly his own needs as well as convey an underlying message that he feels he needs to be listened to.

It may be that the carers will be asked this opening question if the client has difficulties with comprehension, but the information it provides is invaluable in terms of focusing on therapy goals.

Goal for the session

Getting the clients to measure their criteria for success within a session, as well as looking at the outcome of therapy as a whole, is good practice. They will begin to notice for themselves the changes they are making towards finding a solution and not be dependent on what the therapist determines as measurements of success. It also allows for the SFBT belief that every session can be seen as the last; at the end of the first session practitioners will usually tell the clients that they would like to see them again and hear about what is going better, but in later sessions they ask clients whether they think they need to meet again. 'Such questions begin to send a message to clients that they are competent to decide what is best for themselves' (De Jong and Berg, 2002).

Useful starting questions are:

* What are your hopes for the session?
* How will you know this session has been useful to you?
* What will it take for you to say it's been worthwhile coming here today?

The reply may be one that looks more like a miracle and may mean that you don't do 'the miracle question', which will be explored later in this chapter. Clients who stammer, for example, may say 'I'll feel more confident.' In SFBT you want concrete, achievable goals, but it may be at this stage that clients are unable to translate feelings into 'doing things'.

Above all you are looking at the clients' language, and noting down what they say to feed back to them as a reminder, or to pass on to others. Their own words can be much more meaningful to them than ones chosen by you. You are not training to use a model here. You are developing your listening skills and your ability to notice, in collaboration with the clients, the potential solutions to their problems.

The miracle question

'The miracle question is a central intervention in the solution-focused repertoire' (O'Connell and Palmer, 2003). Hypothetical solution questions – imagining what life will be like without the problem – are not new in the world of therapy, but the power of the miracle question was discovered accidentally by Insoo Kim Berg in the early 1980s.

She asks the question slowly and gently, using frequent pauses to allow for the clients to absorb what is being said, and the effect is quite mesmerizing. Video recordings show that many clients break into a smile and their eyes light up as they begin to describe in detail how their lives will be transformed.

> Now, I want to ask you a strange question. Suppose that while you are sleeping tonight and the entire house is quiet, a miracle happens. The miracle is that the problem which brought you here is solved. However, because you are sleeping, you don't know that the miracle has happened. So, when you wake up tomorrow morning, what will be different that will tell you that a miracle has happened and the problem which brought you here is solved? (de Shazer, 1988, p. 5)

Clients respond in various ways to this question. It's not easy to make a leap of faith and imagine how your life will be changed when the problem is solved. Give them time. Wait in silence. If clients say 'I don't know', wait a bit more for them to come up with a more complete answer. Usually prompting clients with 'Guess!' gets them going, as most people are able to guess at something.

Another response is the 'pie in the sky' pipe dream. Cecil is 68-years-old, lives on his own, has a stammer and suffers from moderate/severe PD. His answer is as follows:

Cecil: I would bound out of bed. My hands wouldn't shake and I could write letters and use the telephone well. I'd go to restaurants and be able to manage a knife and fork, and people wouldn't look at me.

The therapist compliments him on being able to visualize the miracle day so clearly, and together they look at what part of that miracle day he could realistically be doing now. She treats what he has described as the means to something else rather than as an end point:

Therapist: So you'll be using the telephone and going to restaurants. What difference will that make to you (and others)?

The miracle question is a very powerful tool for Cecil in that it enables him to realize that he is still the same person, despite the disease; he enjoys writing, eating out and taking care of his appearance. He is able to address some of the isolation he is experiencing at home, and begin to communicate more effectively with others.

The miracle question has a future focus and is a tool that helps clients identify what changes they want to see in their lives. For that reason, many practitioners use it towards the beginning of a session, so that they can follow with exceptions (to look at when parts of the miracle is already happening), and scaled questions (10 represents things that you do on your miracle day). Sometimes clients need a little more time, through exceptions and scaling questions, to make a shift from thinking only about the problem to focusing on solutions. If this is the case the miracle question can be worked on towards the end of the session, at home or in the next session.

Asking the miracle question does require confidence and practice, and training is needed to ensure that maximum benefit is ensured.

Other practitioners of SFBT prefer to frame this key goal-setting question in a different way. You can talk about a pill or magic wand (good for children), or avoid such words as 'miracle' or 'magic' altogether. Asking clients 'What are your best hopes from our work together?' or just 'Suppose for one minute that the problem has gone', gets them to think of their preferred future. A client may be dying, but they can still have a future focus, even if that future consists of days rather than months or years.

Exceptions

Traditional practice states that you do an assessment or case history before effective therapy can proceed. SFBT questions the format of some of these as it is easy to make a person feel worse at the end of a history-taking session. However, SFBT practitioners are not 'history-phobic', and with documentation becoming increasingly important to protect yourself against accusations of malpractice your flexibility depends on the situation in which you find yourself. This will be discussed further when looking at outpatients in detail in Chapter 3.

A SFBT assessment does not usually search for causes or antecedents to the problem in the past (Cade and O'Hanlon, 1993) but is oriented towards the present and the future (what the clients do not like in the present and what they want to change in the future). Information about the present is elicited through asking questions about the times the problem does not happen, or happens less, and the ways clients have of coping with set-backs or continuing difficulties.

An exception may not be immediately related to the problem that brought them to the session. If the goal is to feel more confident, then regardless of whether the issue is stammering or slurred speech, the exceptions will be looking at times when confidence is improved in all areas of life. Permanent body injuries cannot be undone. However, finding out when clients are managing situations better, and identifying good coping strategies, has always been the task of the therapist. The key is to enable clients to see that an exception is not a fluke; if it has happened once it can happen again.

> Once exceptions (and/or hypothetical solutions) are seen by the client to make a difference and are seen as associated with the goal, then the present is clearly salient to the client's future and the client's task becomes the arduous one of making the exceptions into the rule (de Shazer, 1988, p. 191).

The important thing about exceptions is that they are not remarkable or unique – they are happening all the time. Recent exceptions are the most useful as it is all the more plausible they could happen again. In the case of clients who have suffered a stroke, they can start noticing from the time of onset to when you see them; even if there are severe speech difficulties, there may be times when they, or their family, feel that things are slightly more successful. Once an exception has been identified, the therapist needs to mine it for details, as the more detailed you get, the more grounded in everyday life experiences the exception becomes. The wh-questions are used – who, what, when, where – and most important, 'how'.

Notice that 'why' is not included. You do not need to know why the clients problems are occurring before you can help them. A grounding in medicine will help you understand a disease better, but the assumption in the problem-solving approach that there is a necessary connection between a problem and its solution has led to the belief that different diseases require different treatments, often without allowing for the clients' perceptions about their problems and solutions. In SFBT you do not view yourselves as expert at scientifically assessing clients' problems and then intervening. Instead you aim to be expert at exploring clients' frames of reference and identifying those perceptions that clients can use to create more satisfying lives (Berg and Reuss, 1998).

Questions to elicit exceptions

- *When* does x occur less/never?
- *Where* does x occur less/never?
- *Who* is around during this time?
- *What* do other people notice about you during this time?
- *How* do you make these things happen?

The question 'How come?' can be used instead of 'Why?' so that we ask:

- *How come* you're able to do that?

The following case example illustrates some of the points made above. Peter is a 69-year-old man, with a history of TB and shortness of breath, who has been referred for an assessment of his swallow. He complains of difficulty eating and drinking and no abnormalities have been detected on a barium swallow. A bedside assessment of his swallow shows that he has a tendency to gulp his fluid, maybe as a result of his claim that he used to be able to down a pint of beer in six seconds!

Therapist:	When do you notice the eating and drinking works well?
Peter:	When I'm not stressed. If I take my time then everything works better.

The therapist is able to work on this and, within one session, feels that Peter is sufficiently aware of safe swallowing strategies for him to be discharged. An advice sheet is given, but he has already outlined for himself half of what is written on that sheet. The outcome was a truly collaborative way of working; a solution-building approach.

'Noticing' is a key word in SFBT. It is about the therapist/nurse/doctor noticing statements clients make about what they want different, and what the clients have already tried to improve their situations. It is about clients noticing what they are doing when the problem has less control over their lives. This shift in perception towards the construction of a solution, rather than the deconstruction of a problem, is the fundamental difference between the SFBT and problem-solving approach.

One therapist comments that she constantly uses the question 'What have you found that works?' at home as well as work, after she was trained in the SFBT approach. 'Even that one question makes all the difference. I do it unconsciously all the time now. It moves away from me just telling people what to do straight off.'

Scaling questions

A study done on carers of people with non-acute dysphasic and non-dysphasic stroke found the following:

> Generalised self-efficacy is the belief in one's ability to perform a behaviour and carers who scored higher on this scale had lower levels of distress ... the severity of emotional response to the illness is more likely to be affected by the perception of the disease and the coping strategies used rather than the presence of the disease, and this should be taken into consideration when providing services. (McClenahan and Weinman, 1998, p. 142)

In order to elicit clients' strengths, and get them to self-evaluate complex, intuitive observations with regard to anything from confidence levels to motivation, scaling questions are an extremely useful tool. Typical scaling questions in SFBT would go something like this:

- On a scale of 0-10 with 0 being the worst that things have been (for example, when you came into hospital?), and 10 is how you want things to be, where would you say you are now?
- On a scale of 0-10 where 0 represents you have no confidence that things are going to improve, and 10 represents you have a lot of confidence that they will, where would you say you are now?

These two questions are good starting points. The first question could have 10 as the day after the miracle, if the clients have already described the preferred future. The second is a good indicator of their mood; following on from looking at exceptions, they may already perceive things as more hopeful than when you first met them.

Consider the following case example of 49-year-old Frank who has a stroke while at work. He has a wife and young children, and it is devastating for him; although his comprehension is unaffected, he wakes up in hospital to find that he is only able to communicate effectively by writing. The therapist asks him where he feels he is between 0 and 10, drawing a line for him to mark on a piece of paper (which she does with every client to keep in her records and for them to mark themselves in each session). Frank is so enthusiastic with this idea that for the entire duration of his stay in hospital he is able to offer specific examples of progress, as he perceives it, on his own copy of the scale, even after speech greatly improves.

Frank finds that he likes to scale in percentages. The first three days are indicated well below his 50 per cent mark, with no specific percentage given each day. He is, however, very clear about progress made within the 50 per cent mark. When first seen, Frank is able to see that he has moved from no speech to being able to make a phone call and buy something off the hospital trolley. Day 2 is marked by a long-distance phone call, and that he was able to say 'B' more easily.

Day 3 notes
I can blow up my cheeks
I had 4 visitors
I feel more in control of my life
I don't feel embarrassed
Fed up with writing so much.

There are no right or wrong answers to scaling questions. The numbers themselves are fairly meaningless, and if clients place themselves at a 7 when they still have marked difficulties with speech, then 7 it is. Frank wrote on his piece of paper 'Effective communication is not dependent on speaking alone!'

The real therapeutic power of a scaling question is revealed by the open-ended follow-up questions (Sharry, Madden and Darmody, 2001).

Follow-up questions

- How have you managed to get this far?
- What will you be doing differently when you move up to number x?
- What will your family notice you're doing differently when you're at number x?
- What else will you be doing?
- Are you aiming for 10, or will you settle for something less?

The answers to the last question are interesting. Someone may give 10 as representing 100 per cent recovery of their speech and language after an acute event; even if the therapist thinks this is unlikely, it does not have to be an area of concern. (In fact, at the Chelsea and Westminster Hospital it has been found that frequently clients say they will settle for less than 10, or that they begin to realize that 10 = effective communication/independence, which may not be 100 per cent recovery of speech and language.) What you need to develop as a SFBT practitioner is a 'not knowing' approach, where you do not presume to know what the clients' criteria for success is. Frank decided that when he reached his 100 per cent it would mean he was able to write a letter to the Stroke Association giving his story, and that he would also like to make a speech to his colleagues on the same subject. These were realistic goals, and showed that he recognized the value of specific activities to aim for.

What is important for the clients is the perceived gap between what can be accomplished and what cannot, and in some studies of quality of life with dysphasia the perceived fulfilment of desires had the highest association with interpretations of health and well-being (LaPointe, 1999).

It is sometimes helpful to have more specific scales. If someone wants to work on reading, writing or mobility, for example, with 0 being that there has been no progress made and 10 being there has been 100 per cent progress, you can ask the client to measure change from where they feel they are on a scale by asking the question: How will you know that things are moving forward?

Scale lines can always be changed and modified, as we will see in later chapters. They can enable people to see that life is on a continuum and to be able to measure progress in small concrete steps.

Feedback

The end of a session is just as important as the beginning. You want it to end with an upbeat note and a feeling of having accomplished something, as well as some concrete plans for what is going to happen next. Difficulties will be acknowledged again, skills and strengths highlighted, and attention will be paid to any signs of change in the direction of the preferred future.

Some practitioners in SFBT take a break of 5–10 minutes before giving clients feedback. This is particularly advantageous if the session has been monitored from behind a one-way mirror, when others are able to add to the list of compliments or any clients' solutions that you may have missed. Usually the break is for quiet reflection alone.

Leaving the room may not be possible if clients are unsafe on their own. On the ward in hospital, you could find that leaving the bedside is an invitation for someone else to step in and start something else.

The advantage of writing down clients' key phrases during the session is that they are easily accessible. More importantly, they are the clients' own words, so that compliments can be focused on the clients' strengths in language that is meaningful to them rather than empty praise from the listener. An example of this is the client with physical difficulties mentioned earlier (p. 6):

> *Therapist*:   I would like to say again how impressed I am that despite all the difficulties getting here, you persevered. You told me that you're stubborn, determined and organized, and I can see that these are very useful strengths in helping you move forward.

Most clients are not expecting an affirmation about what they want and what they are doing that is useful to them (De Jong and Berg, 2002). More often than not, it is apparent that they are pleased.

To link the compliments to the concluding suggestions or tasks it is useful for the practitioner to say 'I agree with you that ...' For example, in feedback to Cecil (p. 8), the therapist might say 'I agree with you, Cecil, that being able to use the telephone well and enjoy eating out are important goals. You like being with people, and it's not fun feeling that they're all looking at you in restaurants. Therefore, I suggest that ...'

Here some 'homework' may be set. Typical observation tasks are simply noticing any improvements and what clients are doing to move up the scale. Cecil may be asked to pay attention to those times when it feels like the telephone calls have gone better; what he was doing then, and who he was talking to, so that he can report back the next session.

Behavioural tasks require clients to actually do something. They are based on information gathered during the session and are actions the practitioner believes will be useful to the client in constructing a solution. Cecil had mentioned that sitting on a high stool by the bar in a Spanish restaurant recently had meant that he wasn't stared at as he got in and out of a chair, and he had been able to eat *tapas* with his fingers. The therapist encouraged Cecil to continue to look for places where the environment was helpful to him.

Before they leave, clients are asked:

*   How has the session been useful to you?'

You will note that the practitioner does not ask, 'Has this session been useful to you?' There is the assumption that clients will be able to identify what has been useful, and they often come up with a surprise answer. Whereas you thought you had been talking/working on x, they say they enjoyed working on y. It enables clients to think about what they have got out of the session and links in with the question you ask at the beginning ('What do you hope to get out of this session?'). Did they meet that goal, or did it turn out that something completely different was more useful to focus on? It is a question clients can continue to reflect on once they leave the room, and it can provide some sort of closure.

Clients are asked when they want another session. More on the length of time between sessions, and the number of sessions in total, will be covered later in Chapter 3.

Key points in first session

- Problem-free talk
- Problem definition
- Goal for the session
- The miracle question
- Exceptions
- Scaling questions
- Feedback

Subsequent sessions

At the Brief Family Therapy Center they have developed the acronym **EARS** to show the cyclical process of interviewing recommended to the practitioner. Your role after the first session is to help clients identify exceptions and explore them in detail.

E stands for eliciting the exception. You will start the subsequent sessions with:

* So, what's better since I last saw you?
* What's different?

If the answer is the same or worse, then it may require some persistence, but the majority of clients will be able to identify exceptions. You will see in the case examples later how to deal with situations where clients have deteriorated, using 'coping questions'.

A refers to amplifying it, by asking what is different about this exception time and how it happened:

* How did you get the idea to do this?
* Who else noticed this change?

R is reinforcing the successes and strengths. Complimenting is useful here:

* That's quite an achievement.
* How come you were able to do that?

S reminds you to start again:

* What else is better/different?

Using the **EARS** technique reminds you of the core concepts of SFBT. You are looking at what is working well in the present, and taking time to acknowledge steps made by clients towards finding solutions in their lives. You are reinforcing the idea that they are using existing skills and resources to achieve this progress.

Rather like learning the piano, where finger techniques are taught before reaching the next level, questions to elicit exceptions, scales or a miracle are just techniques to help develop a collaborative approach between clients and the therapist/doctor/nurse. It is assumed that clients often know what is good for them, and just need more encouragement to notice this and do more of it.

This chapter may give the impression that the SFBT approach is mechanical; a sort of recipe book where there is a question for every occasion. The phrasing of questions is precise, and some people do write these on a prompt sheet when they start. Maybe the last word here should go to the clients. Invariably they don't pinpoint the actual method but just comment on how it works, as they become aware of their achievements.

Key points

- Look for what works rather than what doesn't work (problem-free talk)
- Encourage clients to clarify their own goals (preferred future)
- Work on clients' strengths rather than weaknesses (exceptions/scales)
- Amplify and reinforce positive change
- Use feedback to summarize points covered in the session

Summary

SFBT enables people to shift from looking at their disabilities to focusing on their level of health. Practitioners can help clients realize their strengths and resources to reduce the impact of any problem on their lives. Beginning with the first session clients are facilitated in defining for themselves what they see as their goals; the miracle question is one way of clarifying the preferred future, with exception-finding and scaling questions being used to help measure the level of success. The practitioner uses the clients' language for feedback, and on-going work between sessions is encouraged. The methods involved in solution talk will lead you to discover clients' hopes for the future in a way that is simple, effective and, in the majority of cases, brief.

Chapter 2
Clients in the acute setting

It may be assumed that because of poor health, particularly in the acute stage post surgery or when clients have suffered a neurological event such as a stroke, it is not possible to work with the SFBT approach. At present, many doctors, nurses and therapists spend a considerable amount of time focusing on the details of the trauma, and only follow problem-oriented treatment plans. Clients can feel that they have lost control of their lives, and the hospital becomes the centre of their focus.

Yet as with any crisis the situation will usually stabilize. SFBT helps clients to focus on the future as well as the present, so that discharge planning begins on admission and the real world beyond the hospital walls becomes the focus. You can work with any clients as long as they or their carers can define a goal, however small; solution-focused procedures are as useful to clients in hospital as to anyone else.

Following the introductory chapter with a discussion of the acute setting has been done for a number of reasons. First, it is a reminder that SFBT is more an attitude than techniques that a practitioner has to follow. Time constraints or client fatigue may mean that you are able to give only small bursts of input, and the first session format is quite different from the one already described. Looking back, however, you are able to identify the subtle ways in which the approach has influenced your work and how your questions are phrased differently. Even though clients come in to the hospital as an emergency and answer numerous questions on admission, which are asked all over again by different staff when admitted to a ward, it is probable that they are never asked the question, 'How will you know that things have improved?' If clients are too unwell, carers could be asked this question or, 'How does x usually handle difficult situations?' The effect could be to help normalize the situation and target clients' resources, as well as obtain useful information for those caring for the clients in hospital.

Second, if the hospital treatment planning uses a problem-oriented framework that emphasizes assessment of symptoms, diagnostic classification and evaluation of outcomes specific to the diagnosis, you will need to decide how much initially you feel you are able to incorporate SFBT into your work. It may be more a question of integrating new skills with existing ones. You may not be able to change a diagnosis of cancer, for example, but how the client progresses from there depends on a number of factors. Case examples may help with this by looking at what a diagnosis means to clients, how they can look for signs that mean the diagnosis is less or more relevant to their life, and through examining the questions help them decide what they want.

Last, the hospital environment offers good examples of how important it is to listen to clients. You are not going to rush in with goaling and solution-building without first having heard and acknowledged clients' pain in distressing circumstances, but there are always opportunities to reflect back strengths and discover possibilities as to how to move forward.

This chapter will look at a variety of clients with communication and swallowing difficulties; some may have minor concerns, others are dealing with bigger issues such as those found in palliative care. Working with students is also included in this chapter, as acute hospitals can be seen as difficult placements, and SFBT can be helpful in changing this perception.

The acute hospital: advantages and opportunities

Kay Vaughn and colleagues, working with inpatients at the Colorado Psychiatric Hospital, point out that SFBT is consistent with the aims of nursing interventions: it builds clients' trust, promotes their sense of control and positive orientation, affirms and supports their strengths, and sets health-oriented mutual goals (Miller et al., 1996). Many occupational therapists already see recovery as the development of a desired lifestyle rather than symptom removal, which fits in with SFBT where the way forward does not depend on a reduction of the problem. Work can start with any client from the first meeting, even if the client has not chosen to see you. Probation and child protection services are obvious examples of involuntary clients, but we could also include here some clients in the acute hospital.

Jonathan, a 50-year-old man who has suffered a stroke, is someone who never presses the call button for assistance, does not want to be seen by anyone, and refuses to be shaved by the nurses. As his appearance deteriorates he is increasingly perceived as a 'difficult patient', 'very depressed' and someone who should be considered for anti-depressants and psychiatric help. So someone tries something different; they ask him the question 'I can see that you want to be left alone … what is it that is important to you about being left alone?' It turns out that he wants to do things himself and feel more in control, and he has decided that being able to shave is one of his goals. Nobody has asked him previously what his goals are or how he perceives his recovery. A short while after this he manages to shave himself, and he then goes on to discuss the miracle question!

> New ideas peculiar to solution focused brief therapy itself include the disconnection between problem and solution, faith in the competence of the client and the lack of a formal theory of change. (Macdonald 2004)

The following is a list of ways in which SFBT can be helpful to the practitioner in the acute hospital.

Change

Change can be rapid in hospital. You may find that clients have changed dramatically since they were last seen and any recommendations made are no longer relevant. SFBT helps practitioners feel that by working in collaboration with the client they are always up-to-date with what is needed. You can say:

*   'I can see you've made a lot of progress since I last saw you. How have you managed that?
*   What can I do that's helpful to you now?'

Discharge

Therapists can find it difficult to discharge clients from their caseload when they are still in hospital. The last question, 'What can I do that's helpful to you now?', gives clients the opportunity to say that they no longer need to see you and, if it is appropriate, for you to agree with their judgement.

Assessment

There is a lot of assessment in hospital. Information is gathered on pathology, deficits and risk factors; symptoms rather than strengths. One woman who was being assessed for a rehabilitation unit commented, 'I hadn't realized how bad it was.' If she had also been asked questions on exceptions to her problems and what the next small step towards her goals might be, then she might not have felt so discouraged.

Power

Hospitals are given magical powers. Clients usually believe that things will change from the time of admission, and this fits in with the SFBT belief that change is constant. However, they are in an artificial environment, and SFBT also encourages clients to think about life outside of the hospital, about work and leisure activities as well as their families and friends who can help with goal setting. A question that can help with this is:

* 'Suppose it's the day of your discharge, what will you be doing/planning?'

Problems

There may be multiple problems. In many cases clients can make informed decisions as to what they see as the most important goal. This is consistent with care aims and achieving a successful outcome; if clients are seen as experts on their problems it allows them to take a more active role in their recovery, rather than waiting for professional experts to make decisions for them. You are still the expert in facilitating the change, providing information and making suggestions. An example of client choice is a man who is given lip and tongue exercises to help with speech intelligibility. He decides he feels 'silly' doing these and wants to focus on hand exercises instead, as he has reduced leg and arm movement as a result of his stroke. He agrees to monitor the times when his speech is working better and he discovers that this happens later in the morning, which is useful information for the multidisciplinary team. Furthermore, SFBT helps him work on his mood. When he first comes in to the hospital he says, 'I give up.' Not long after he is able to say, 'I'm not the man I used to be. I need to adjust to the new person.'

Language

Use the clients' language. Because you note down what clients say, this can be a great help when writing in the medical notes, and will often receive more attention than your own comments.

Abilities

Clients who are experiencing severely diminished physical and/or mental abilities need every help and support to recognize change. If change is slow, then SFBT can help show that even the smallest improvement can be the difference that makes the difference. However, the miracle question and finding exceptions may be too abstract for someone with comprehension difficulties. If even scaled questions are difficult, then clients may be unable to actively engage in goals so as to achieve progress or carry-over from therapy. It is hard when therapists have to explain to carers that they feel ongoing therapy would not be productive. SFBT helps therapists point to any progress made, and engages carers in noticing any changes in the future that would necessitate a change of plan.

Trauma

Trauma represents change; crises can be reframed as occurrences or opportunities. While it is helpful for clients to vent their anger, fear and grief, actively probing them for emotional responses may not be following their natural inclination as to how much and with whom they want to talk. Indeed, literature on the immediate aftermath of trauma now suggests that 'professionals should take their lead from the survivors and provide the help they want, rather than tell survivors how they will get better' (McNally, Bryant and Ehlers, 2003). SFBT views the emotional responses as valid and reasonable and a means to something else the clients really want; Jonathan (p. 19) is angry and frustrated because he feels everything is out of control. As soon as he is able to *do* something that is meaningful to him rather than be asked to talk about his emotions (which in all probability he would have refused to do), the level of frustration is reduced.

Key points

- The practitioner and the client notice the small steps
- SFBT can give relief to continuous assessment
- The client is encouraged to think of life post-hospital
- The client can play a part in the decision-making process
- The clients' language becomes the area of focus
- SFBT translates feelings into actions

Focus on the language

Preferred future

Just as we have been looking at clients' perceptions, it is useful to look further at our own perceptions. One could assume, for example, that techniques such as the miracle question or searching for exceptions are not possible if clients have just been admitted to hospital. The hypothetical question may need to be scaled down. Using the example of Jonathan, perhaps the miracle is that the client wakes up the next day and starts to put his life together:

Therapist:	Let's imagine that tomorrow turns out to be a good day for you. How will you know that it's going well? What will you be doing differently?
Jonathan:	I would jump out of bed, kiss the nurses, and go back to work!
Therapist:	What could you do now that would enable you to feel better?
Jonathan:	I would help those in the ward.

Jonathan's first answer is consistent with his desire to be well, in control and feeling some respect back in his life. Within a month he has moved on a scale from five to eight, and his speech is 98 per cent intelligible.

The more you ask questions about the future, and discover how clients are able to describe and enjoy thinking about things in life other than the problem, the less you become fearful of using clients' imagination in order to facilitate change. If the likely outcome is that they are going to leave hospital without the problem being resolved, such as lasting limb weakness or speech impairment, then the following question can be asked:

* How will you adapt to it in a way that brings out the best in you and your family?

Key point

■ Notice your own use of language. It is not that SFBT is a totally new and different therapy; emphasis on efficiency, clear goals and present-future focus is something that all the clinical specialities involved in hospital treatment would recognize. What may be different are the kinds of questions you ask and the language you use.

The focus of the client

Again, the example of Jonathan can be used here. In Chapter 1 the avoidance of the question 'why' was mentioned. If someone had asked Jonathan, 'Why aren't you letting anyone help you?' it would probably have forced him to justify himself, and be followed up by someone trying to persuade him to change his mind. Asking 'What is it that is important to you about being left alone?' acknowledges that he must have a good reason for wanting to be on his own. Agreeing with his perception is not the same as condoning it, especially if he puts himself or others at risk on the ward. People in hospital cope with their environment in different ways and they may believe that acting in such a way is helpful to them, so it can be usefully explored for solutions. Using a SFBT technique, nurses could do scale work with Jonathan; 0 represents him remaining unshaven, and 10 means he could shave himself, so that a compromise is reached as to how he could reach his goal, initially with assistance, yet still feel he is in control.

Another example of the importance of respecting and working with the clients' viewpoint is the case of Robert. As a result of a second stroke he requires a lot of assistance with everyday needs, is unable to sit out in a chair, and has slurred speech:

Therapist:	You look much better today.
Robert:	I want to get out of hospital!
Therapist:	Good ... so our goals are the same ... we both want you to be able to leave hospital. On a scale of 0–10, with 0 being that you're not ready to leave at all, and 10 being that you are ready, where would you say you are now?
Robert:	10!
Therapist:	I think you may have a way to go yet! What can you be doing to get to that position?

Robert, like Jonathan, has strong ideas on the best way to deal with a situation. The therapist knows that he is used to public speaking, and asks what strategies he has used in the past to project his voice. He replies, 'I concentrated on something in the distance and shouted at it!' As he is in a side-room the therapist encourages him to practise shouting; the result is a stronger voice (not strained as in shouting) which he achieves by maintaining a better posture, since he imagines he is speaking in public. It is an example of a client using existing strengths and his own key word (shouting) to help himself do something different. An expert in voice might actively discourage shouting, and go into a long explanation as to how it is harmful to the vocal cords, without first exploring what the client means by 'shouting'. Exploring and affirming clients' perceptions is a major part of what is done in SFBT.

Rephrasing

It is not uncommon in hospital for clients to talk only about what they do not want to continue happening; 'I don't want to be thinking about this all the time', 'I don't want to be getting the words wrong when I speak to the doctor'. A useful word here is 'instead', so that you can say, 'So what do you want to be doing instead?' When clients are encouraged to rephrase what they have said, it can be the first small step towards noticing when this might already be happening. Another word much loved by Insoo Kim Berg is 'suppose':

* Suppose you don't think about it all the time ... what will you be doing?

This can also be used to great effect when someone says 'I don't know' in response to the miracle question. You can pause and say:

* Suppose you did know ...!

One woman responds to this, after initially saying she has no idea what would be different after a miracle has happened, by saying, 'I'd stop shouting at the nurses.' That word 'shouting' again! When the therapist asks what she would be doing instead, she replies, 'I would speak more slowly, and be more patient.' She does not need to be told by the therapist how to begin work on her speech, which is difficult to follow at times.

It is impossible to list here all the ways in which you can adapt and rephrase your own and clients' language to help focus on what they want and thereby facilitate change. It is not that you are trying to trick clients, or

> that one is attempting to do something to someone else with some unstated agenda of one's own. Of course, our agenda is to help our clients reach what they want – their goal or their solution. If it becomes apparent to us that the client wants something we do not do or cannot provide, then we say so and sometimes end the therapy. (Walter and Peller, 1992)

Being precise in how you ask a question elicits a more specific response; it is often the details that are of most use to clients, and a hypothetical question in the present can help identify times when the preferred future is already happening. Unlike exception-finding, this has the advantage that it may have no connection to the problem. Jonathan's route to working on his speech and improving overall began with an action (shaving) and his desire to be independent.

You will notice many examples in this book of questions about future changes beginning with 'When ...', rather than 'If ...', and the present or future tense of a verb used rather than the conditional 'would/could'. For example:

Client: If only I could feel better and more relaxed, I'd let friends come to
               visit me instead of telling them not to come here.
Therapist: So you'll be seeing more of your friends when you feel more
               relaxed. What difference will that make to you (and them)?

These questions simply reflect an attitude of mind; they are reinforcing the belief that change is continuous and constant, and that clients are part of that process. Practising this use of language is an important part of any training in SFBT. Used everyday in the work environment it becomes automatic, so that attention can be focused on listening to the client, their perceptions, and their own use of language.

Solution focused language

- What will you be feeling/doing *instead*?
- What *do* you want to feel/be doing?
- *Suppose* you ...
- *When* will you ...?

Eating and drinking

In 2001 the Stroke Association commissioned the College of Health to carry out a large-scale survey: a total of 2252 clients and carers returned a postal questionnaire, which formed the basis of a report on the perception of care available to people affected by stroke (Kelson, Riesel and Kennelly, 2001). Some of the questionnaires were completed by relatives or carers on clients' behalf, but most of them were by the clients themselves, the majority of whom were admitted to hospital; included in the list of problems as a result of their stroke were 41.9 per cent who said they had difficulties with their swallow.

If you add to this number other clients who have swallowing difficulties as a result of brain injury, chronic disease, cancer or HIV, it is evident that there is a large population of people in hospital who are not managing to eat and drink effectively.

These clients are an important part of the speech and language therapy caseload in an acute hospital. They vary from those who may have minor problems with their food or drink, which may or may not resolve quickly, to those who continue to experience major difficulties long after admission. Regardless of the underlying pathology or the severity of the problem, the impact on clients' lives can be enormous when mealtimes, or even the management of their own saliva, become an issue. SFBT can influence how practitioners assess and monitor clients, as well as influencing clients' perceptions on how their case is being managed. Half of those in hospital as a result of a stroke felt they needed psychological help but did not receive it. Timely access to support is essential.

Assessing and complimenting clients

George has a long history of swallowing difficulties. He has undergone investigations by a throat specialist, and has had a bedside swallowing assessment. Neither of these show any abnormalities, so he is seen for a videofluoroscopy; the X-ray reveals some minor problems, but George continues to be anxious about the fact that sometimes he experiences 'choking and coughing at mealtimes'. He says this has gone on for decades. The therapist is impressed by how he has managed to live with this for so long:

Therapist:	How have you managed to cope with that?
George:	I have to accept it. I know I have to be careful, so I try to drink slowly.
Therapist:	That's a good strategy. It can really helpful to do that.
George:	I'm a patient person and seem to be adaptable. I haven't let it get me down.
Therapist:	Have you always been a patient person?
George:	Yes. When I was first a seaman I used to be seasick ... but I got over it!

The conversation moves away from the problem, with George discussing his past sports activities and achievements. He is able to give himself 8 on a scale (how he feels he is managing his swallow), and once the therapist is happy that he is aware of various safe swallowing strategies, he is discharged.

Like Peter in Chapter 1, SFBT is incorporated into the assessment of a client's swallow. It can be used in a similar way when monitoring clients in hospital; their perception of how they feel they are managing is always a good starting point. Of course there are danger signs with a swallow that clients may not be noticing, which may require an expert to recommend an alternative route to oral feeding. An interesting footnote to George's case is that he displayed marked hesitancy and delay in his speech when talking with the speech and language therapist. He made no mention of this to the therapist at any stage, despite being given ample opportunity to do so.

There are likely to be other areas like swallowing where the attitudinal issue is frequently not addressed. It is hoped that the example of George shows that it does not require additional input of time; indeed, SFBT helped both George and the therapist move towards a satisfactory outcome, in a case that might have otherwise proved inconclusive.

Assessments can include questions that draw on clients' strengths and past successes. Noticing these, the practitioner can compliment clients in a way that is reality-based, and help reinforce in the clients' mind what they want to achieve. When complimenting was first introduced at the Brief Family Therapy Centre, compliments were mainly used at the end of the session; they are now generally used throughout the session, and can be described as either direct, indirect, or self-compliments (De Jong and Berg, 2002).

The conversation above with George shows some direct complimenting, when the therapist reacts positively in response to George's idea of drinking slowly. An indirect compliment is a question that implies something positive about the client. An example of this would be the client with a diagnosis of HIV who said:

Client:	My condition varies. Sometimes I'm really tired and my speech is slurred. If that happens, I choose words carefully and say shorter sentences. My swallowing can be difficult too.
Therapist:	When are the times when the swallowing is a bit better?
Client:	When I keep my head down and concentrate.
Therapist:	How did you know what to do differently? Does it surprise you that you're able to come up with all these ideas?
Client:	Yes, I suppose it does. I'm taking more care of myself and don't want to get tired out. But I've always tried worked things out for myself. I've recently found out that if I dunk my biscuit in the tea, I don't cough with the crumbs.

A self-compliment, which is also demonstrated here, can have a powerful effect on clients. It may be the first time that they have become aware of their own resources, which is a valuable skill in hospital where so much is done for 'the patient'.

A comment that is frequently said at the end of a SFBT session is, 'It's good to know I'm doing the right things.' Clients have the opportunity to list some of these things themselves, rather than the therapist doing it for them, so that when they are given a written handout (as is often the case with swallowing difficulties) the recommendations appear more familiar.

Key points

- Eliciting skills promotes more direct and indirect compliments for the client
- Self-compliments can have the most powerful effect on a client

---

Coping questions

What if clients are so overwhelmed by the trauma in their lives that surviving from day to day is all they seem capable of doing, and looking for exceptions does not feel appropriate?

Consider the two cases of Valerie and Evelyn, both admitted to hospital with swallowing and communication difficulties. Valerie is 80 years old and has suffered a stroke, which she describes as 'devastating'. Evelyn is 67 years old, and has had Parkinson's disease for a number of years.

Valerie is able to identify times when communication is working better. Sunday is a good day because 'I can go to Mass, nice friends visit who don't talk too much, and the ward is quieter.' She describes a vivid picture of what the preferred future will look like, and uses a scale to measure improvement in her speech; beginning at 1, when she has to repeat most sentences so that people can understand her, she moves to 2 (repeating half of her sentences), then 4 (repeating a quarter), and then 6. Interestingly, at 6 the focus is not on her speech but on other things that she is doing such as getting out of the hospital in a wheelchair, and being able to walk down the corridor. Her speech was so difficult to understand when first seen that she was given an electronic communication aid, but this is soon discarded, and she is finally able to reach a number 9 before being discharged.

Evelyn, on the other hand, is quite unable to identify any times when her situation is improved:

Therapist:	When do you feel your communication is working a bit better?
Evelyn:	I don't get much opportunity to talk. I've never been good at it.
Therapist:	If you were to rate it from 0 to 10, with 0 being things were awful and 10 was pretty good ... where would you be?

Evelyn:	At 0. It's difficult ... I'm stuck in a chair.
Therapist:	I'm sorry to hear things are so difficult for you. How have you managed to cope in such difficult circumstances?
Evelyn:	I don't know ... I don't like people treating me like a baby. At the Day Centre they would compliment me on filling in one or two words in a crossword puzzle ...
Therapist:	What would be the best way to show them that you're not a baby?
Evelyn:	They could wait until I've completed the crossword. If people talk over my head I say 'Meow!'

The situation at the Day Centre is a good example of how a compliment can be perceived as unhelpful if it is only motivated by a desire to be kind. Complimenting Evelyn on how she is managing to cope appears to be more successful. At least that is what the therapist thought, until she sees Evelyn on another visit to her bedside and asks her where she feels she is on her scale:

Evelyn:	–10!
Therapist:	So things feel worse ... What would be different, though, at –9?
Evelyn:	I don't know ... I have been at 1 in the past.
Therapist:	Really! When was that?
Evelyn:	When I'm with people ... with the group [Bible discussion group]. I feel I belong. I'd like to be useful to other people. I'm intelligent – I have an IQ of 153!
Therapist:	Wow! How do you show people that you're so intelligent! It's important to show people that just because you've got Parkinson's disease, you're not stupid ... how do you do that?

Evelyn says she is going to think about that. The next visit reveals that she is still at –10. The therapist decides to ask her another coping question:

| Therapist: | How come things aren't worse? |
| Evelyn: | I keep myself busy. I read. I would like to be more mobile. |

Evelyn's responses suggest that her evidence for progress does not allow her to notice any difference from one day to the next. The therapist persists in her belief that change is occurring all the time and that eventually Evelyn will see when some of her hopes are realized. This proves to be the case. When the therapist next visits Evelyn she seems more cheerful, but would still only allow herself –9:

| Evelyn: | Two medical students came today. It's the second lot I've had ... |
| Therapist: | See how you've been helpful in hospital! Some people tell them they don't want to be disturbed! |

Evelyn is beginning to sharpen her awareness of what she is already doing to cope with her situation. Despite feeling 'stuck' and overwhelmed, she is well enough to be helped out of her bed in the morning into a chair, and she is willing to spend time talking to others. If she manages to move up to 1 again she can be complimented on that also.

Coping questions

- How did you manage to get out of bed today?
- How have you managed to move all the way from –10 to 1?
- What would it take to go up just another half-point to 1.5?
- What will you be doing then that you're not doing now?
- How optimistic are you that if things stayed the same that you could manage?
- How have you coped with things in the past?

Palliative care

The experience of many practitioners who work with the terminally ill and use SFBT is that the methods and techniques can be used to great effect without the need to make too many adjustments. There are the coping questions mentioned above, which could also include:

* How have you managed to keep going [in the hospital/hospice]?
* Have you surprised yourself with how you've dealt with it?
* How will you know when you're dealing with it even better?

Clients in palliative care are simply people with a future to face that is limited in nature. It is possible to ask the miracle question without being fearful of the response; practitioners find that clients do not reply that their brain tumour, for example, has gone, but are able to focus on what they want to do with the rest of their lives. A possible way of asking it might be:

* Imagine, the day after you die, whenever that is ... days, months, years ... you're looking back and discover that you're pleased with all the things that have happened between now and then ... what will be telling you that it went well?

Dominic Bray, a clinical psychologist in oncology at the Royal Preston Hospital, gives the example of a client who reframed this question by saying 'I've been thinking about that ... you mean "When I'm on my deathbed, what will I not be regretting?"' (Bray, 2003).

He has also used this question with relatives:

*   When x dies, whenever that is ... days, months, years ... what will you be looking back on and saying 'I'm glad we did that' or 'We did the right thing by x'?

Swallowing difficulties can give rise to ethical dilemmas with regard to nutrition and hydration. One such case is Ken, a young man with a diagnosis of HIV, who has a fluctuating level of alertness and is at risk of aspiration; his mother is aware that he is coughing on teaspoons of fluid, but feels that oral intake 'is one of the few pleasures left to him'. It is eventually decided that artificial feeding via the stomach is the best option, and his mother gives mouth care only as his condition deteriorates. She is able to identify, however, that she 'has done the right thing' for her son in the last few months leading up to this point: 'Over Christmas I was able to give him small amounts of his favourite things to eat and drink, and he enjoyed this.'

Within the palliative care setting clinical staff, as well as families, can find their resources being challenged in order to deal with the multiple physical symptoms that are often accompanied by emotional, cognitive and sensory changes (Brajtman, Azoulay, Gassner and Yeheskel, 2002). SFBT principles can help manage some stressors in this environment by encouraging a collaborative approach within staff supervision:

*   How will you and you colleagues know when you're doing your job especially well, and in which ways is this already happening?

Two case examples are now included to put SFBT in context and give a clearer picture of how help is provided over time in the hospital setting. As you would with those who may not be near death, you need to use your skills to help clients discover their own way forward.

Case example: Graham

When his condition suddenly deteriorates as a result of HIV, Graham is admitted to hospital and referred for help with his speech. He is 45-years-old and has been working until the point of admission. When the therapist first meets him, she asks him to scale himself from 0 to 10.

Graham:	Last Thursday I wasn't making sense at all. I couldn't answer the phone or write a fax. It's very frustrating – one day you can speak the next you can't.
Therapist:	What have you found helpful?
Graham:	Slowing down. First thing in the morning, I'm relaxed. At the moment I'm at a number 5 ... I would normally be at 8/9. I want to

go on working. I realize I can do less now. I need to get my head round it though. I know I can't go on working from 6.30 in the morning to 7.30 at night.

A week later he says:

Graham: I will have to give up my work, which is difficult for someone who has been independent all his life.

When asked about his speech he is able to say that 'I know if I can't find a word it's no good getting stressed about it.'

The following week Graham has a temperature and is finding it more difficult to speak. When asked about where he is on a scale of 0–10 his response is not what the therapist expects:

Graham: Number 8. If it is ordained that this is the way I go, so be it. I want to die at home.

He is able to go home for the weekend, and tells the therapist, 'I've done everything I need to do.' Graham is discharged some time after this.

About two months later Graham is re-admitted to hospital, following a course in radiotherapy which has resulted in weight and hair loss and 'non-fluent speech'. Comprehension continues to be good.

Graham: Words ... stuck. My wife ... tomorrow bring notepad. Can't say word. Today better. Last week terrible. Just sat there.

Graham is given an electronic communication aid and visited the next day. There is some improvement, and he is able to identify that he has been in a low mood recently:

Graham: And me ... normally cheerful. Difficult home ... couldn't do things. Embarrassment ... useless. Need feel useful.
Therapist: How can you be feeling useful now?
Graham: Write letter daughter. Sort out money things.
Therapist: Anything else?
Graham: Can use e-mail. Can't work again. Not used to it.
Therapist: What could you be doing instead?
Graham: Could help friend at Muslim centre. I go to hospice next week. Time to think. Wife finds it difficult. Not a problem for me, dying. Will happen when it happens.

Graham later decides that he does not need the communication aid. SFBT helps the therapist feel that she has done all she can regarding speech and language, and that it is appropriate to discharge.

Case example: Francis

Francis is 80. He has advanced prostrate and bone cancer, and has been referred for help with his swallow as he is 'only managing to eat and drink very small amounts'. A bedside assessment reveals that there is no abnormality with the swallow itself. He tells the therapist he is holding water in his mouth

Francis:	... because my mouth is dry. I've never eaten or drunk very much. I don't enjoy eating and drinking.
Therapist:	Is there anything that would make a difference here with the eating and drinking?
Francis:	No. I don't think so.
Therapist:	If you were to think of one thing that you enjoy eating, just a little more than the rest ...?
Francis:	The pudding perhaps. It indicates the end of the meal.
Therapist:	So you prefer sweet to savoury food?
Francis:	No. Not really.

The therapist could have left at this point, having done her swallowing assessment and discussed soft consistencies that Francis could choose from the menu. However, she notices that his voice quality is poor, and decides it might be useful to do a scaling question to see if he brings up any issues to do with communication:

Therapist:	On a scale of from 0–10, with 0 being things aren't too good and 10 being things are going pretty well, where would you say you are generally now?
Francis:	*(immediate response)* About 2.
Therapist:	So ... I know you've been in hospital for a while, and things aren't much fun being stuck in hospital. You could have told me 0. How have you managed to be at a number 2?
Francis:	*(voice quality changes)* It's about getting out there and doing it. I've been trying to keep myself occupied.
Therapist:	What are you doing to keep yourself occupied? Do you listen to the hospital radio or watch television?
Francis:	No. I don't like the radio or television. I sometimes write. See if you can find a red notebook over there ...

It transpires that Francis has written a very funny piece on 'The hospital gown and hospital beds'. It is a short insightful piece ('How can these open-backed, ugly gowns be liked by anybody but the medics? Why is it that hospital beds always have thin blankets and leave the feet exposed at the end?') and written in beautiful handwriting (of which the patient is also proud). The notebook is buried under a pile of things and inaccessible in his side locker; it is extremely unlikely that the therapist would have 'happened' upon it, or indeed felt able to pick it up and quiz Francis on its contents.

The scaling question has provided a way forward. Francis fatigues easily, and what follows is a fifteen-minute exploration of how he feels he is best communicating now. He mentions that he feels his voice quality has changed but that he is not overly concerned with this. He makes no mention of his disease or the prognosis.

Francis is retired. He spends time at home writing the occasional piece for publication, and drawing cartoons. The cartoon in his notebook on bed tilts is very amusing, and he has drawn some other cartoons for the ward a few months previous over the Christmas period. The therapist notes no entry over the last month. Is it something he is going to do? Maybe a new entry would be a step forward; a 2.5/3?

Francis' condition has deteriorated rapidly by the following week when the therapist returns, and his daughter is by the bedside. He is no longer eating and drinking, but further assessment is not appropriate. Remembering a comment by a colleague whose father has recently died in hospital ('It was good when people took the trouble to pass by and say hello'), the therapist tells his daughter how much she appreciated Francis sharing the contents of his notebook, and how much they had laughed about hospital gowns and tilt beds.

Before using SFBT the therapist would have felt empty-handed, with nothing to offer the family but platitudes. Instead there was something specific to share, as a result of one short session. It gave the therapist the confidence not to be overwhelmed by the daughter's grief, and to do something different other than leave the ward without contact. There was some sort of positive outcome for the therapist, and more importantly, the possibility that this was the case for the daughter too, however small.

Key points

- Identify what's working, however small
- Discover what the client would find helpful to move forward
- Work on the clients' goals
- Being solution focused promotes confidence in the practitioner
- SFBT helps focus on a positive outcome

Students

The above case example helps demonstrate that the needs of the practitioner are often no different from those of the student; that by focusing on the clients strengths, they will be guided as to the way forward, and that by asking themselves the question, 'What did you learn about your client and yourself today?' the possibilities for learning is enhanced.

SFBT can help practitioners supervise students, as well as help students monitor themselves. On the first day the supervisor can ask the students to rate themselves on how they feel about hospitals, with 0 being they find hospitals difficult and 10 being they are comfortable in the hospital environment. From 0 to 10 how confident are they that they can improve on this? This gives valuable information to the supervisor and a good baseline for the students to return to some weeks later.

Some of the points listed below give further ideas that may be helpful for students, with particular reference to the acute setting.

Role play

There are times when it is not possible for students to get direct contact with the clients; an example is when they are not yet trained in the necessary skills to carry out an assessment and can only observe the practitioner. Rather than learning through discussion, SFBT is experiential in nature, which means it is ideally suited for role-play and pair work. Many placements are now for at least two students, so this should not present a problem.

Solution talk

The practitioner can indicate that the focus of supervision is on solution talk, not problem talk. Clients in the acute setting often have multiple problems, which can be confusing for someone who is not used to the sheer volume of information. One student agreed to feeling 'a bit muddled' after describing her session with a client to the therapist.

Therapist:	I think you may be right. So how could you do things differently? What else could you be doing?
Student:	Well. Doing it, but making it shorter. I think I tend to put too much down and ask too many questions.
Therapist:	Yes. I think that's a good idea. It can be a bit overwhelming for me too if there's too much material.

Resources

The students can be given the opportunity to identify their preferred way of learning when asked,

*   'How have you successfully learnt new things in the past?'

It will reinforce the view that they are already competent in dealing with new situations and that they have resources which will be useful to them now. This is the goal of any SFBT training, and is worth remembering in unfamiliar settings such as hospitals.

Level of competence

By identifying 'What am I doing right?' the student can go on to decide that they need to do more of what works. Even if initially there are only small examples, increased feelings of competence will lead to other successes and change. This is known as the 'ripple' effect.

Self-monitoring

SFBT encourages the belief that change is constant and that no problem remains the same; this applies to any issues the client or student may have. Students can use scales to monitor themselves:

Therapist: What are you hoping to get out of today?
Student: I would like to be a bit more independent. Not having to be told what to do, or having to ask to do it.
Therapist: So on a scale ...
Student: 6 probably.
Therapist: What will you be doing at 7?
Student: Well ... probably being able to take the initiative more when seeing a new inpatient. Trusting my own judgement, or not needing to ask x two or three questions on what to do.

The expert

There is no 'right' way to view things, and it is acceptable for students to say to clients, 'I don't know, what do you think?' It is part of the belief that you are not the expert on other people's lives, and underlines the need for students to listen to the client. If they struggle to help clients find their solutions, they can use their supervisor's experience and knowledge to move things forward in the next session.

Becoming more focused

In an attempt to be encouraging to clients in hospital, students can be over-keen to compliment clients on what they do. An example is one student who would always feedback to the client, 'You did really well' when they finished each task together, and it could at times appear patronizing. By learning to be more specific in her feedback, and encouraging clients to self-compliment, the student was on her way to becoming a more effective practitioner.

Jargon

Students appreciate the lack of jargon when thinking in a SFBT way; professional jargon is useful in hospital, but the words of the individual client can often be even more helpful, especially when feeding back to supervisors. So much time can be spent by students worrying about whether they can give the correct name to the clients impairment, and it could be argued that this is something that could be done equally well at college. Noting down the clients' own description and using this to formulate goals and predict outcomes can be harder skills to develop.

Key points

■ SFBT is ideally suited for role play and pair work

■ It promotes solution talk, not problem talk

■ It uses past successes to build on the present and the future

■ Students can learn to notice gradual change in the clients and themselves

■ There is no 'right' way to view things

■ Students learn to listen to the clients' language

■ Feedback will be enhanced

An example follows of how a supervisor and student can collaborate together on a case.

Case example: Sylvie

In her mid-fifties, Sylvie is an independent and active woman. She suffers a stroke that results in total loss of speech, and no movement in the right side of her body. She is in hospital for over five weeks, and is then seen as an outpatient.

A student starts her placement while Sylvie is on the caseload, and helps with assessments that need to be done to measure improvement. Four sessions now follow that show how SFBT plays a part in therapy input.

Session 1: The student carries out a language assessment. When this has been completed the supervisor, who has been sitting in on the session, takes the lead and asks some SFBT questions (the student observes). Sylvie's speech and language has improved greatly but she is concerned that progress is slowing down, and she is also worried that her writing is 'shaky'. Exception-finding questions are used to identify strategies that help things work better;

she decides, for example, that she will tell strangers, 'Excuse me ... my speech isn't so good at the moment.' To monitor her writing she decides to keep a diary.

Session 2: The student starts the session again. Sylvie wants to return to work, so writing continues to be an area of concern, and various functional activities are carried out to practise writing skills. Towards the end of the session the supervisor again takes the lead, and looks at how Sylvie will know when she is ready to go back to work. Scaling questions are used.

Session 3: The whole session is run by the student. A case history is carried out for college, and further work on Sylvie's writing is done. Sylvie says she is going to start work soon.

Session 4: Again, the student runs the session. Sylvie has returned to work; they are able to discuss coping strategies she is using in the workplace, which include getting colleagues to take things upstairs for her, asking for help when completing invoices, and getting the secretary to write letters. Handwriting strategies are also discussed, as well as word-finding strategies (pausing for thought, thinking about the word until it comes back to her and visualization). This is all documented in the notes and fedback to the supervisor later.

SFBT helps the student and supervisor work together to facilitate Sylvie's transition from being 'the patient' to someone who is able to engage in part-time work. Sylvie needs 'functional' work and a 'holistic' approach; work that can be difficult to formulate for a student who is unfamiliar with the problems that arise from a stroke. Through scale work and exceptions, a practical framework is ensured, and one that the student is quickly able to take on and develop.

Six months after this Sylvie has one more session and is discharged. Nearly a year after the stroke, she continues to experience difficulties at work as a result of residual problems. She finds she gets irritable with colleagues, tires more easily, and gets tearful when she is on her own at home.

The 2001 Stroke Association survey shows that 61 per cent of clients report mood swings. A long catalogue of other problems includes aggression, anger, boredom, frustration, loss of motivation, hallucinations, loss of social skills and change in personality. Comments are made such as 'My father was physically OK. It was his mind that had changed. We were told nothing. If this was normal, would it improve, who could help?' or 'It would be helpful if there was someone understanding that a stroke victim could talk to about their problems following stroke. I was so depressed because I felt no-one understood that I contemplated suicide and phoned Samaritans.'

Faced with any of the above, it is no wonder that students find their placements challenging. No-one would suggest that it is down to any one person in hospital to deal with all of these difficulties. Indeed, there is a need for everyone in the health care profession to feel they are equipped to respond to these problems in some way. Some would argue that it is not within their remit, and fear that they might find themselves committed to lengthy therapy. SFBT can be a solution: the practical nature of the approach means it can be used within the existing hospital framework yet at the same time 'many clients tell us that we have been talking about their feelings' (de Shazer, Dolan and Berg, 2004).

Care plans, for example, exist in hospitals to provide a framework for improving nurse–client communication, as well as improving communication between nurses themselves. They can be perceived as an extra piece of paperwork that is not relevant to clients' care and difficult to write, especially where emotional problems are concerned. Incorporating SFBT into the overall treatment facilitates the formation of measurable positive goals, and there is the added advantage, that when evaluation no longer relies on interpretation, a nurse who is not familiar with a particular client can still complete the evaluation. Student nurses can also develop from an early stage

> the skills to make the process of paperwork as indistinguishable as possible from the process of helping the individual client. The concepts of brief therapy provide one means of achieving this goal. (Brimblecombe, 1995)

The aim of any team of professionals within a hospital is that they work in a co-ordinated way on goals that are achievable. Clients' perception of treatment can be dramatically improved if, instead of seeing a hospital as a place where all their problems can be solved for them, they see themselves as an integral part of that process. Sylvie is able to leave hospital because of intervention from the medical and therapy team. Her return to work and some sort of normal life is achieved by her own ability to monitor herself and perceive life in a way that highlights her achievements; a skill she develops while using SFBT in hospital.

Sylvie:	I realize how unrealistic I was when I first saw you. I can't work everyday anymore.
Therapist:	So what are you doing with your time instead?
Sylvie:	My goals have changed. I was doing too much before, and now I suppose I'm enjoying London more.
Therapist:	Sounds like you're more relaxed,
Sylvie:	I'm more relaxed. Yes ... I like that word.

> **Key points**
>
> - Clients need to be able to measure change for themselves
> - SFBT helps them see they are coping in a difficult situation
> - Student supervision benefits from a solution focused framework
> - SFBT provides skills for students to monitor themselves and their clients
> - Practitioners can give positive feedback

Summary

Clients in hospital have the same needs as in any other setting; they need to believe they have some control over their environment and they need to have some measure of their own achievements. SFBT helps practitioners look at clients' perceptions and facilitates a way forward, particularly in difficult situations where clients are coping with multiple problems that appear to have no resolution. The focus is on opportunities to reflect back strengths so as to elicit practical and achievable goals for the present and the future. In a environment where there are a large number of professionals making demands on them and performing endless investigations, direct, indirect and self-compliments give clients encouragement. Practitioners can use SFBT techniques to monitor students, and they can also train their students to incorporate the model into their growing repertoire of skills.

Chapter 3
Clients living
independently

As we continue to study how solutions develop, we are concluding that there are more similarities between the treatment of phobias and the treatment of wet beds and the treatment of conflictual couples than there are differences. And I am not sure that these differences make any difference! (de Shazer, 1988, p. 140)

This chapter includes examples of a variety of clients living at home who have self-referred, or been referred by a doctor, consultant or therapist, for an appointment as an outpatient at the hospital. Communication and/or swallowing problems have arisen as a result of a stroke, Parkinson's disease, head injury, learning difficulties, voice problems or a stammer.

Clients may start a session talking about specific problems. However, often you will notice that a pattern emerges, which is that other issues are included that are common concerns seen in any outpatient department. These tend to be psychosocial features such as self-esteem, role change, lifestyle changes and quality of life. Recently 173 speech and language therapists were asked about their experience of the psychosocial impact on dysphasic speakers (Brumfitt, 2003). Twenty-two per cent said that half of their time was spent on psychosocial issues, and 95 per cent believed that these issues were 'important' or 'very important' to the clients' overall outcome. Approximately two-thirds of the therapists did not distinguish between the psychosocial effects of dysphasia, dysarthria and dysphagia.

Practitioners also have many issues in common when trying to provide the best service for their clients. What is the best way to make an appointment? How much information is needed about clients before they are seen as an outpatient? How much time is needed for the taking of a case history and assessment? What kind of 'homework' should be given? Should a contract be made with clients regarding the number of sessions available?

> **Key point**
>
> ■ SFBT challenges us to re-consider some procedures and allows us to incorporate new ideas into existing frameworks. This process begins even before we see the clients for their first appointment.

Pre-session change

From the moment when clients decide to come to therapy, whether it is going to the doctor for a referral to a specialist, or picking up the phone to ask for help, small positive changes are occurring. Clients feel that they are doing something about the problem. A. Jay McKeel (Miller et al., 1996) looked at research into pre-session change. One group of clients were asked why they did not attend their first appointment and more than a third of this group said they did not come because of improvements that had already taken place. Another study found that nearly 40 per cent of clients attending their first session at a family therapy centre reported some pre-session improvement in their situation.

In order to strengthen this effect you can invite clients to look out for change when making the appointment:

*   Often between making the appointment and arriving for the appointment people notice change. You might like to look out for any changes.

This could be asked on the phone, included in the appointment letter or in a leaflet. At the Chelsea and Westminster Hospital a leaflet is sent out with the appointment letter outlining SFBT and what will happen in sessions. When clients come for the first appointment they are asked:

*   What changes have you noticed since the appointment was made?

Sandra, a 53-year-old lady with a stammer, says she feels her speech has improved slightly in the previous weeks and that she feels less anxious. A brief discussion follows which looks at the strategies she has been using that have been helpful to her. Coming to see a specialist is sometimes the first time a person who stammers acknowledges it in public. This requires courage and determination: an opportunity for compliments, and seeing their actions outside therapy as a step towards already achieving their goals. Another way of using the waiting time before the first appointment is to ask clients:

* The therapist would like to see you on ... She'd like you to pay attention to what you would like to keep the same in your life between now and when you come for the appointment.

Clients already feel engaged with the therapist, and begin to focus on what is working rather than just the complaint. It can also facilitate an explanation in the first session of the solution focused approach, if it is felt one is needed.

Client focus

Consider the following details given in referral letters to the Speech and Language Therapy Department. They are not unusual:

* Teresa is 31. She has been going to group therapy for help with her stammer where they have been practising 'block modification'. She has also learnt about 'prolonged speech' and relaxation when attending individual therapy in the past. She says 'they didn't really help'.
* Steve has difficulties with his throat, his voice and his swallow. Numerous investigations have been done, including a videofluoroscopy, but nothing untoward has been found. A family member and close friend have recently died, and he is on anti-depressants as he feels anxious and stressed. He has a high profile job.
* Malcolm has been to a reflexologist, faith-healer, and homeopath for help with his Parkinson's disease, as he feels these approaches 'look at the holistic view rather than isolated aspects, as does traditional medicine'. Aged 69, he is anxious and finding it difficult to deal with his diagnosis. He has mild speech problems.

A useful exercise when training in SFBT is to look at what appear to be negative points in a referral and see how you can pull out clues to client strengths and possible solutions. What does the client see as the most important issue? What do you notice that the client has done to move forward? Clients' difficulties can appear complex and intractable: 'A solution-focused approach provides ways of thinking which avoid over-complication' (Winbolt, 2002).

In Teresa's case the therapist congratulates her on searching for what might be useful, and having a clear mind as to what she does and does not find helpful. She explores the helpful strategies that Teresa is already using, one of which Teresa says involves kicking her husband under the table at dinner parties for help when her speech gets into difficulty! Three weeks later, after looking at the miracle question and scale lines, Teresa comments, 'My husband says I look happier. I'm smiling more.' She is able to switch off the answering machine (she would never answer the phone before), and has managed to make a hairdresser's appointment on the phone.

Steve's referral letter makes the therapist wonder how he has managed to keep going despite everything that is happening in his life. When he begins to describe some of these difficulties, she asks Steve to rate himself on a scale of 0–10 in terms of where he is now overall:

Steve:	I'm at –5.
Therapist:	How come things don't feel worse than that? You could have said –10.
Steve:	–10 would be suicidal. My Dad and my sister aren't ill. The anti-depressants ... they're double dose ... they're a temporary solution.
Therapist:	It sounds like you have good coping skills.
Steve:	Life has knocked me down often and I've picked myself up.

Using the miracle question Steve begins to think of all the things he would do without the problems: 'I'd have lots of energy, do the washing, go swimming, buy my friends presents'. When he is asked how the session has been useful he replies, 'I will see what things I need to do and what things I don't *have* to do.'

Not long after, the therapist receives a letter from Steve saying he has decided to see a psychotherapist. He has realized that the problems are lifestyle issues rather than difficulties with his voice or his swallow. Although he is seeking help from yet another professional he is focusing on his own strengths and resources more effectively, and beginning to engage in activities that will enable him to take control of his life.

A similar case is Venetia, who was referred with 'oedematous arytenoids, acid reflux, coughing and false cord phonation'. Numerous visits to health professionals over a long period of time do not appear to have helped with Venetia's symptoms, and she has been seen in the department before. However, enabling her to see how well she is coping, and focusing on what *is* working, appears to set Venetia on the road to recovery. It also allows the therapist, within a relatively short space of time, to tell Venetia that she does not need to come for further therapy. This is empowering for both practitioner and client, and leads to a productive outcome as a result of looking at a 'difficult outpatient' in a different way.

> We (disabled people) have to gain control of our own lives, our own physical rehabilitation, our own personal assistance. (WHO 2001)

Motivation

Venetia is perceived as a difficult case because nobody can establish exactly why, for example, she is coughing all the time. By taking the focus away from the cough the therapist is following the SFBT principle of doing something different. Similarly, this approach can be used when clients appear not to cooperate with therapy, and an example of this has already been given in the previous chapter (Jonathan, p. 19). It is not uncommon for practitioners to receive outpatient referrals such as this regarding a 42-year-old lady with voice problems:

> Mary has been given jaw and tongue exercises to help with her hyperfunctional dysphonia. She has been practising diaphragmatic breathing and exercises to reduce hard glottal attack. She has found most of these exercises difficult to carry out, and has usually attended her next appointment stating that she has been unable to do the latest exercise. No significant progress has been made.

Mary confirms this when she is first seen, saying she does not have time to do the exercises. Working with scales, the therapist is able to offer Mary a way of monitoring herself so that she can decide how she moves from 2.5 (her current position) to 7.5/8 (where she wants to get to).

Practitioners need to assume client competence. They need to believe that if they are told there is no time to do the exercises that either (a) this is the case, or (b) clients have a good reason to believe that these particular exercises are not helpful to them. Rather than assume that these clients are not motivated, the way forward is to listen to what has already worked in the past, ask for their definition of the problem and what they might want.

In recent years de Shazer and others have adopted the assumption that '*all* clients are motivated for *something*' (George, Iveson and Ratner, 1999). It is not useful to divide clients according to different levels of resistance or non-compliance, which has originated from a medical model of helping people influenced by Freud. More helpful is the belief that if clients have agreed to speak to you, then you will find the clients' competences by asking questions that help clients articulate what they actually want. Because the emphasis is on the preferred future, the clients' view of the problem is taken into account but is not the focus of therapy.

* What do you want to come out of this hour/this meeting/this conference?
* What will be helpful to you?
* You must be doing something right. How did you get out of bed this morning?

Five months after his stroke Andrew is back in hospital as an outpatient requesting further assistance. He says that he was told he was 'cured', but that he doesn't feel that he is. He has mild naming difficulties, difficulty writing, and a 'variable voice'.

It is unlikely that Andrew was told that he was 'cured' but this is his perception, and it is the therapist's task to help him think through what is best for him and his own treatment. This is what emerges in the first session:

* Andrew's social circle doesn't feel that he is different to how he was before, but this is not how he is feeling inside: 'I don't always understand complex questions and I get tired when speaking.'
* His preferred future is being able to 'talk freely and be more energetic'. He wants to go to exhibitions once a week, go shopping and play the piano as he did before the stroke.
* When encouraged to look at times when the 'miracle' is already happening he admits that he is already playing the piano, going to exhibitions (once a month), reading, walking and swimming. Andrew says at the end of the session 'I will notice what I'm doing right. I can also see that tiredness is not abnormal.'

Andrew could have been another 'difficult' case: looking for his definition of 100 per cent recovery in speech and language would have been a lengthy and possibly fruitless task. Only focusing on his mild impairments may not have highlighted the fact that at home he is doing a lot to help himself feel reconnected with the outside world. Indeed, he is later able to admit that although he is making mistakes on the piano, 'I'm able to tell myself that maybe I made the mistakes before the stroke. I've come out of a dark tunnel and I'm happier with myself. I'm trying to see what makes a difference. I don't feel I need to come again.'

Again and again the comments of those engaged in SFBT are that 'I'm more accepting of myself' or 'I seem to be able to look forward now, not back all the time.' Hence the point made at the beginning of this chapter: although there can be different physical and cognitive changes as a result of stress, disease or a neurological event, clients often come for help with the same underlying issues. All they might need is reassurance that they are doing everything they can to reach their optimal level of independent functioning. SFBT is not a 'cure' for dysphasia or dysphonia, but there is a good chance that it will enable clients to meet their goals more effectively.

Key points

- Change happens from the point of referral
- Both the practitioner and client need to look out for that change
- Even the most negative referral holds possible solutions
- Assume that the client knows what is helpful to them
- SFBT gives the client reassurance that change is possible

Taking a case history

Certain medical information needs to be included in a referral letter to ensure good management of care. A voice referral, for example, will need to include information from the Ear, Nose, and Throat (ENT) clinics regarding the health of the larynx.

However, unless clients feel the need to give every last detail of the problem, this is not essential to effective therapy. Practitioners are open to what clients choose to tell them. If clients immediately launch into a detailed history when first seen, it might be useful to stop them for a minute and say:

* I have some of the details already – what do *you* think is important for me to know?

Insoo Kim Berg (SFT listserv, 2003) gives the example of someone at the other extreme: a lady comes into the clinic and says she refuses to talk about her problem, but that she is in need of a solution. They are able to look at solutions, and she leaves the session satisfied. Insoo does not need to ask about her past or what the problem is (although it is usually clear from the solutions what the problems are).

This requires a significant shift away from a lot of material currently being used; the completion of lengthy case history forms is frequently seen as the first step of treatment. Information is gathered, a treatment plan is made and intervention is given. Practitioners using the SFBT approach may find certain aspects of this record-keeping irrelevant to their work and working against their belief that they are co-participants in solution construction. Andrew's first session is a case in point. He is asked for his goal for the session, his preferred future, times when this is already happening, and how he feels the session has been useful. There is no need to complete a case history form as ample information is elicited for both parties to work on. Andrew moves back and forth between problem talk and solution talk, and is asked for clarification if it is needed.

What if there are agency documentation requirements to get information for initial assessment and treatment plans? For necessary identifying information a brief questionnaire can be completed before seeing the practitioner. If history-taking can only be done in the session, then a task can be set at the end that will focus clients' attention towards solution building for the next session. Another option is to include competency based questions when collecting history data, such as:

* You couldn't speak at all when the stroke first happened. How did you manage to cope with that?
* You've had all these problems with your voice/speech yet you've held a steady job for most of your working life. How come you've been able to do that?

Inviting a narrative with 'How come ...?' or 'You must have a good reason to ...?' can be more informative than who/what/when type questions.

Key point

■ Paperwork that more closely follows the stages of solution building is replacing some traditional problem-focused documents, and includes goals and hopes for the future, past successes, strengths and coping strategies, and feedback.

Progress notes can be organized around scaling with space to record details, such as what needs to happen for clients to move up the scale. Kay Vaughn and colleagues modified all their documentation systems to reflect their changed philosophy of care in a hospital setting (Miller et al., 1996). In-house training can help medical staff to consider integrating new skills with existing ones, even if it is only to suggest that doctors ask some solution focused questions when meeting with clients. Collaboration between doctors and those working with SFBT at primary care level can help avoid referrals to health services in secondary care (Wales, 1998).

Assessment

John is 68, and has difficulty processing information as a result of a traumatic brain injury (TBI). An assessment shows difficulties with activities such as sequencing and verbal reasoning, and although he is performing at a 'high level' the assessment is long, so that there little time left at the end of the session. The therapist finishes with her usual question:

Therapist: How has this session been useful to you?
John: It's been absolutely no use whatsoever!

How useful it is to get feedback! The therapist has forgotten to put the information in context. She has not reminded him at the end of the session how the information would be useful to her, or how John could use the information for himself. Furthermore his family do not appear to find the information useful either, despite the therapist's attempts to put the findings into a functional framework.

In the next session scales are used to help John establish for himself where he feels he is in terms of improvement. He places himself at 6/7. When asked how confident he is that he will be able to improve on this he says 7/8. Then he realizes that 10 does not mean 'difficult', and he repositions himself at 2.

Therapist: How can you move a little up the scale and feel more confident about things?

John: If I had a bit more consistency.

It is not entirely clear what John means by 'consistency'. However, the therapist feels she has gained a considerable amount of information from the scales that she could use to work on with John and his family. First, there are pointers as to John's level of insight and mood. Second, it is evident that working on levels of confidence would be useful, and it is unlikely that the assessment helped with this. Third, he is encouraged to see for himself that he has improved since the accident first happened and that 6/7 is quite an achievement. Fourth, the therapist and the family are able to discuss the meaning of 'consistency'. The therapist suggests that it might be the need for John to feel that the day is following some routine, as he is complaining of too much going on and things being out of his control. The family are pleased to work on this and report back.

Scales show times when a preferred future is already happening, provide details and a description of any improvement, and prompt questions as to how the improvements have been made. If progress is minimal then the focus can be on times when the problem is less acute, or looking at how clients have managed to persevere both now and in the past. The 'flow' of a session (Iveson, 2002) allows for information gathering to be constant, without the traditional demarcation between case-history taking, assessment and treatment.

Of course standardized assessments are important in order to establish a baseline for treatment or therapy and as a guide to when discharge is possible. They are essential for research and measuring outcomes. No one assessment can truly claim to cover all areas of communication in sufficient depth, and what is being suggested here is that SFBT provides techniques that can be a useful adjunct to the way you work. 'Although solution-focused brief therapy is a treatment in its own right it can also be used to complement other treatments' (Iveson, 2002).

One client commented: 'I liked that last session – the miracle question made me feel warm inside, and makes me look at the practical side.' Because the practitioner is looking at what makes clients more hopeful they frequently describe their experience of solution focused work in this way. SFBT does not, however, theorize about internal or interpersonal psychological states. Indeed, there are those who believe that the 'therapeutic relationship' is not a necessary part of successful therapy (George, 2003). It is the questions that are crucial, rather than the person of the questioner. If you believe this it can feel strangely liberating; you feel more comfortable writing down key comments during the session, for example, rather than worrying that this will detract from how the client interacts with you. Knowing what to do with clients' answers is the mark of a good therapist.

Some case examples will now be given to illustrate how SFBT can facilitate change with different client groups seen in the outpatient department. It is important to bear in mind the following points.

Religious/cultural differences

It can be hard for some Muslims to answer the miracle question or to use self-rating scales. If their situation is 'God's will' then searching for improvement may not be the way to deal with issues, unless it is looked at from a different perspective. Sometimes practitioners ask:

* What would God notice you doing differently?

Uniqueness

There may be 'typical' SFBT techniques, but clients' responses to them and their solutions are unique. There can be no list of questions to ask for every occasion, just as there are no 'right' or 'wrong' answers.

Change is continual

It is the clients who are doing the work; a session may only last one hour but clients will be changing all the time away from the therapy room. So you can ask:

* I haven't seen you since x. What's different from when I last saw you?
* What in the last session did you find useful in the days/weeks between sessions?

Key points

- SFBT helps measure the clients' level of insight and motivation
- Solution focused work facilitates the negotiation of goals
- SFBT can be used as an adjunct to, or replace, some existing assessments
- The practitioner and client look for evidence in signs of actual behaviours
- The time between sessions is important

Language again!

It has been suggested that for some people who have difficulty understanding spoken or written words as a result of a stroke or a TBI, for example, the preferred future or scales are not useful tools to works with. Damien, aged 28 and recovering from a severe brain injury, is able to work with the miracle question with assistance from his girlfriend who attends the session. What seems to be more meaningful to him however is a scale that is asked in a deliberately 'open' way:

Therapist: Compared to where you were before, where are you now and where do you want to be?

Damien: I want to feel safe like I used to.

Therapist: When are the times that you feel safe at the moment?

Damien: When I'm at home. Going out in the street doesn't feel safe as I might have another [epileptic] fit. I'm not cooking 'cause I might drop the frying pan.

The management of Damien's case, as with so many people in his situation, is to do with finding areas of independence to build on. The therapist is able to work on his scale of 'safe' so that he is be able to get out more and achieve his goal of attending a social skills group. He also identifies past strengths:

Damien: I'm good at art – I used to draw graffiti on trains!

Charles, who has residual problems following a stroke, is another person who finds specific words useful. When asked the miracle question he says:

Charles: I wouldn't feel so isolated ... such solitude.

Therapist: What would you feel instead?

Charles: Tranquillity.

Six days later the therapist gets a phone call.

Charles: Is that x? Tell me the word that we discussed!

Practitioners working with children and adolescents find that looking at 'sparkling moments' (White, 1995) helps identify the times when the preferred future is already happening. It can also be a useful phrase for some adult clients to help them identify exceptions.

Try something different

Quite often clients have developed a strategy that is unhelpful to them but they are convinced that they should try and try again until it works, instead of doing something different. This is suggested to a man with memory problems who keeps 'getting lost' trying to find a word, so that he then also forgets the question. He decides that he's going to just 'leave it and move on'. His confidence that things will continue to improve moves from 6 to 8.5/9. He begins to ask himself the question 'What could I do differently?' When he is in a dinner party and can't follow the conversation, he tells himself that he can ask people to slow down and give him more time to respond.

Another client, with severe speech problems two years after her stroke, also finds this approach useful. She used to look at when she *wasn't* achieving her goal of maintaining eye contact for 30 per cent of the time. Encouraged to look at the times when she is achieving it, she is then able to clarify what exactly she is doing right so that she can do more of it: 'It works better at nightime. I'm relaxed. Maybe it's also that the muscles that push my eyes to the right are tired.' Her communication overall improves, until the session when she spends the time talking about parenting issues rather then her speech. The therapist feels she is able to be discharged from the caseload.

More scales

There are many different ways of working with scales. With children you can use play dough to demonstrate the size of a problem, or get them to do a walking scale with paper plates. Moving up a scale can be measured in behaviour or pictures rather than words, while colours may also be a good indicator of change. SFBT scales have no fixed points, so they can be infinitely variable.

Some examples are given here of clients who are very precise in their use of scales.

Clara has mild Reinke's oedema, marked glottal chink, and fluctuating voice loss. She is aware that stress, as a result of poor sleep, anxiety about her family and general health issues, is affecting her voice badly. She is given advice and information on the vocal mechanism and hygiene, and works on a reduction of laryngeal tension. SFBT looks at the time she is achieving a 'good' voice. She starts to notice that instead of getting 'pain and hoarseness' once a day, she can go two to three days without these symptoms.

Her scale becomes one which measures how she is moving from 0, which represents her as an 'ill woman', to 10, which is Clara as a 'well woman'. By the time she gets to 8 after five sessions, the pain she had in her hand and her throat has gone and she is off painkillers. She has also achieved another goal that is to get her husband to book a holiday. Interestingly, she began therapy not wearing any jewellery, and she has now begun to put on earrings. She says her measurement of how 'well' she is relates to the amount of jewellery she wears. Those familiar with Personal Construct Theory, used by some therapists working with people who stammer in particular, will see similar threads here (Hayhow and Levy, 1989).

Another client, who has a severe stammer both in his mother tongue and in English, finds it difficult to identify the times when his communication feels better. This phrase 'better communication' can be too broad, as he may miss the potential of the times that he is doing something that leads to this end state. The solution, however, is in looking for exceptions, and he mentions the phone calls he makes to his mother: 'inside of me is very cold. I am relaxed'. It is true that the client sweats profusely at the beginning of the session. The therapist, however, decides to start by focusing on the times he is already relaxed rather than beginning therapy by teaching him relaxation skills. Gradually the client notices other times when he is nearer to his goal of 'cold'.

One of the many advantages of building on existing skills as opposed to having to learn new ones is that the role of the therapist, or a 'programme', becomes less central to success. A study on the experience of adults after therapy with prolonged-speech (PS) found that these novel speech patterns, as with most behavioural treatments for stammering, not only fail to eliminate stammering but also '*exacerbate* the feelings of being different that adults experience' (Cream et al., 2003). As one participant commented, 'normal people' don't use fluency techniques. Furthermore, if their use of PS is ineffective, it is felt to be due to their lack of skill and diligence rather than any shortcoming of the therapy programmes. The authors conclude that the challenge is to integrate the use of PS 'with a range of other skills and strategies clients may already have'.

The difficulty can be identifying these skills and strategies. Scales can be used to chart progress in a person's life, and they help maintain the focus on the client rather than on how others need to change for 'the problem' to go. One 22-year-old who is sent by his father for help with his 'social talking' comments that his own speech is fine, but that it is his father's communication that needs help. SFBT uses the clients' own language; this young man works with computers, and he is able to see that change in only one area can make a difference, and that several small steps move towards a workable programme.

You can work on several scales in one session. Towards the end of the session the client can consider,

* What might happen to one scale as a result of an improvement on another?'

so that multiple problems, which appear to be hopelessly interconnected, can be seen together in a constructive way.

Stuart is 20 and has not eaten solid food for three years, but there are no physical signs as to why he should feel his throat is in spasm. Scales look at what he is already eating, which is mashed potatoes, cauliflower cheese, yogurts, cream cheese, cakes, egg yolks (not the white) and chocolate (which he melts in his mouth). Scales help him measure how he can move up a point with different consistencies until he has gone from 2, when he began therapy, to 5 (eating sandwiches). Although he is identifying his strengths as he moves up the scale, he is still focused on the problem, and it may take a considerable amount of time for him to feel he is eating a 'normal' diet. Change in the other areas of his life is the difference that makes the difference. He begins to go out with his friends, starts a carpentry course, starts driving lessons and generally feels more confident. 'My throat is feeling easier and not seizing up as much as before. I'm hungry and enjoying my food.' Eating is no longer an issue.

The unexpected

A therapist who works with the SFBT approach is having a discussion with a nurse specialist in palliative cancer care. The therapist asks whether this client group could ever use self-perception scales to measure change. She is told that this would be a bad idea because, as treatment is not working, there would be a negative outcome.

It is hoped that some of the ideas already mentioned in this book might suggest a different outcome. Be prepared for the unexpected! If there are concerns regarding people with physical difficulties that are not going to improve it may be useful to do the following: ask these clients to draw a line between the part where there can be a workable solution and the other part where, so far, there is no workable solution. Another idea to help with a similar scenario might be:

*   How much of feeling better is your doing?
*   How much of feeling better is medication? (Berg 2000)

Injections into the vocal cords to help with voice production or medication for Parkinson's disease, for example, is an aid not a cure. The real 'feeling better' is up to the clients to work on, whether it be meditating, eating well, deep breathing, being with their children or going out to work.

Cecil (already mentioned in Chapter 1) who has PD is an example of the need for the practitioner to have an open mind. One might assume that as the disease progresses, clients will feel more and more restricted in movement and communication, in fact in all aspects of their lives. Cecil, however, is able to identify some sides of PD that have been a positive advantage. Having been a fiercely independent and private man he is able to say: 'I have become friendlier with people. I am talking more, relying on them more and asking for help.'

Cecil comes back for a session two years later. He feels his speech has become more difficult due to 'tightness of the mouth', and that his 'thought processes' have deteriorated.

Therapist:	What helps with the tightness of the mouth?
Cecil:	When I'm relaxed. In the morning, for example. I do feel stronger though. The consultant is pleased with me ... but I want peace of mind.
Therapist:	What will help you achieve this?
Cecil:	If I do more activity. Or if I had one person with me who I can talk to, and who can communicate with me.
Therapist:	Who's helpful to you at the moment?
Cecil:	The consultant – I have confidence in him. My accountant is honest and reliable. My masseur and cleaner are reliable and genuine.
Therapist:	Having confidence in people is obviously important to you.
Cecil:	Yes. And the masseur helps me with things too. But then I have to listen to her talk about her husband and kids.
Therapist:	When do you have peace of mind now?
Cecil:	I've bought a video. I've watched *Citizen Kane* about 70-80 times! I appreciate its use of language and camerawork - I wanted to be a film director once. I also enjoy books ... Proust, for example. I listen to talking tapes.

Cecil is able to focus on what is working for him, and is able to appreciate others. His scale of how he feels he is managing has improved since he was seen two years previously.

Other examples of the unexpected can occur when people talk about their miracle day. One man who comes to therapy for help with his stammer describes his miracle day as being able to talk on the phone 'smoothly', being calm and able to concentrate, taking out the rubbish, cleaning the bath and hoovering the carpet. After the first session he goes home and does the housecleaning: 'I felt I'd done something,' he tells the therapist. Times when the miracle is already happening have the advantage that, unlike exceptions, they are not related directly to the problem.

Another man talks about how his stammer interferes with his work, and that the miracle would be doing good presentations. The first session is spent on this topic. At the next session he surprises the therapist by saying, 'I know it's useful talking about it [stammering]. I never have before. After the last session I spoke with my wife about it for the first time.' It is likely that presentation work is always going to be difficult for this client. Therapy is determined by what he feels is the next step, rather than the therapist planning the course of the session.

The miracle question can trigger thoughts and events that do not manifest themselves immediately (Burns, 1999). It may be a small event in the clients' lives that becomes meaningful. An Italian lady who has vocal nodules and a loud voice, which she is trying to monitor more effectively along with issues of anger and stress, says, 'If you are happy inside then if people are rude it doesn't matter. I love what I do. Yesterday a lady came to work and I could have sold her a more expensive bag, but I felt it didn't suit her. I can't sell a little woman a big bag. Then I love myself.'

Feelings of frustration, anger and sadness may always continue to affect clients' lives, or for long after the health care professions have withdrawn from a case. James gets frustrated when reduced understanding as a result of a stroke means that he can find everyday activities challenging. He is, however, learning to monitor himself more effectively:

James:	I'm learning how to use the computer. It's difficult! I've decided not to do it at all for a week.
Therapist:	So you're taking a rest.
James:	Yes. I'm having a rest. I haven't been painting either.
Therapist:	You're making choices.
James:	Yes. I can choose to leave ... not to do something. I can be quiet. Yesterday I used my bank card in the ... [unable to find the word]. I wanted some money. My card disappeared in the wall! But I was able to walk off. I can laugh at my mistakes.

James appears to like the words 'choice' 'rest' and 'being quiet', as he repeats them to himself several times. The therapist asks questions that encourage him to translate these abstract states into everyday actions.

Key points

- What can you (the practitioner/client) do differently?
- Existing skills, rather than a 'programme' or medication, are central to success
- Expect the unexpected

Feedback

Feedback is occurring throughout the session. There are advantages, however, in creating space at the end of a session for more formal feedback. This may be organized around (a) compliments, (b) some comments that you would like to say or repeat, from your own experience or research, for example, and (c) a task. If it is not possible to leave the room to collect your thoughts (and allow clients time to think about what has been said), then a quick glance over your notes will help you to pick out key phrases. Some feedback to James is:

> *Therapist*: I'm impressed by how you know what to do when you need a rest. You're doing a lot of things that you weren't doing when you first got home, and that's great – especially learning to use the computer! But progress can be slow, and a lot of people get frustrated after a stroke, especially when they get home and they can't do things as quickly as they did before. I agree that being able to laugh at your mistakes can be very helpful.

Feedback needs to be simple and straightforward; it needs to affirm what clients want and what is important to them. It can highlight recent changes and normalize common concerns. If the clients are doing things that are helping them towards solutions, their task can be to do more of the same. If their solution is less developed, they need to observe the times when things are working well for them. The practitioner can ask further questions in the next session to elicit exactly what it is that the clients are doing in these situations.

There are those who work with SFBT who do not see task-setting as part of their repertoire of techniques and who believe that as the tasks become more important, the practitioner's thoughts and actions become more dominant (George, Iveson and Ratner, 1999).

Although they are not essential, tasks can help remind clients that they are the ones doing the work in their everyday lives and that it is the time between sessions, and long after therapy has finished, which is the area of focus. Asking 'What's different or better?' in the following session will usually reveal whether the task has been done or not.

Tasks are an important feature of Steve de Shazer's work. Choosing the appropriate task can be particularly rewarding for those clients who feel they want to 'do something' between sessions, as they can be more productive than some of the more traditional therapeutic drills or intervention. Some ideas for clients are listed below.

Following the 'if it ain't broke don't fix it' principle, ask the client to:

* Notice what you would like to continue happening in your life.
* Notice what things are working well for you.

Some clients are able to identify the times when things are working well quite easily. Ask the client to:

* Continue to do what works. See if you can give me any more examples about the times when you're doing things that are helpful to you.

If clients are finding it difficult to identify exceptions, do something different. Ask the client to do one of these activities and think of it as an experiment:

*   On the odd-numbered days of the week pretend to feel different and see what happens. On the even-numbered days just do as you normally do (Walter and Peller, 1992).
*   Flip a coin. Heads means you must do an activity that you feel is helpful, tails is just a normal day. Notice what's different on a heads day in your life (Berg and Reuss, 1998).
*   Each night before you go to bed, predict whether or not tomorrow will be a day when [you feel better about your speech/language]. Then, at the end of the day, before you make your prediction for the next day, think about whether or not your prediction came true. See if you can account for any differences between your prediction and the way the day went (De Jong and Berg, 2002).

When clients perceive exceptions as occurring as the result of someone or something else, it can be helpful to modify the basic observational task with an element of prediction, as in the last task given. An example will help put this in context.

Patrick is 27 and has a severe stammer, which he says has not been helped by either individual or group therapy in the past. He is able to identify times when things are working better for him, but feels these are linked to outside influences; when he had a job and money, his speech was much better. He believes that it is therefore unlikely that things will improves significantly at the moment when he is unemployed and feeling 'depressed'. (He did, however, manage to self-refer!)

Patrick says that Saturday and Sunday are always 'good days', whereas Friday and Monday are 'bad days'. When asked to continue to predict his good and bad days, Patrick claims he has been 100 per cent successful. However, he seems to have higher expectations for a better day, and initiates activities that show he is establishing a self-fulfilling prophecy. Furthermore, on closer examination, he sees that good things are also happening on the 'bad days'. He forgets to mention, for example, that he has received a letter on a Friday offering him a job interview.

After five sessions Patrick is happy to be discharged. He still has bouts of depression, and he still has a stammer, but he says his friends have noticed that he talks more, and that he's more cheerful and contented. 'I have the feeling that I can cope and that I can concentrate on when I'm doing things right. I've realized that having a stammer isn't that bad.'

A group of adolescent students with learning difficulties get the encouragement they need to use their resources to be creative from the following task:

> Do something different. It may be something that seems practical and straight forward or it may be fun, interesting, and/or exciting. It might even be a combination of both. Whatever you choose, choose something to do that will enable you to experience even more success accomplishing your goal. (Thompson and Littrell, 1998)

The psychological needs of those with learning difficulties tend to receive less attention than other areas of their lives. Comments from these students in this study using SFBT include: 'I got to talk to someone who didn't tell me what to do or just give me advice.' Furthermore they come up with practical solution-building strategies that the practitioner could never have predicted such as: 'I squeeze my keys when I get mad instead of mouthing off', and the majority of them report positive changes in other aspects of their lives.

Key points

- Use the clients' language to summarize goals
- End the session with positive feedback (compliments)
- Observation or behavioural tasks can be useful

Reports

Details of a session are written in the practitioners' notes and include clients' answers to the miracle question, exceptions, scales and feedback given. Clients may like to take a copy of their scales home so that goals are written down and remembered more easily. Some practitioners send a letter after each session complimenting their clients on their achievements and on being able to move from x to y on a scale.

On discharge, it is required practice to write a letter to the referrer, a copy of which is now sent to the client.

Key point

- SFBT can help give a framework to comments on how improvement has been achieved, and facilitates user-friendly language. Scales can be used to remind clients of progress made.

This is an extract from a report written on Clara:

> Using a SFBT approach, Clara gives her level of achievement as 8 (out of a total of 10), and notes that her confidence is 9 (in that she believes her voice will continue to improve).

More specific information is seen in the following:

> SFBT was used to very good effect to allow Mrs. X to explore her own strengths to overcome this [voice] problem. Mrs. X's difficulties with her voice were mainly due to an inner lack of confidence and resulting anxiety. Towards the end of the session Mrs. X had discovered ways within herself to deal with this.

Another example is a letter to a doctor regarding W, who says that previous therapy 'hasn't changed my perception of my speech'. In one session, the miracle question allows him to see that despite his stammer he could become more relaxed and more spontaneous with his communication:

> W. has been seen for one session using SFBT. He has set his own goals for achieving success namely
> * Putting speech difficulties in perspective.
> * Moving ahead – not holding on to bad feelings
> * Recognizing the importance of body language and improving the skills he already has.
>
> W. will contact the department when he feels that he requires further input.

Number of sessions

As you can see in the last report, the decision as to whether therapy is finished or not remains with the client. This way of working can appear quite different to a system where outpatients are offered a fixed contract, which is frequently given as six sessions spaced over the same number of weeks. You can find in the literature on SFBT that successful studies have followed this format (Cockburn, Thomas and Cockburn, 1997; Zimmerman, Prest and Wetzel, 1998), but everyday practice suggests that there is a variation between one to eight sessions, rarely more than this, extending across several months.

Discharge can be based on 'concrete, behavioural, measurable signs that the client can identify as indicators that her recovery is moving in the right direction' (Berg and Reuss, 1997). Look at the clients' scales regarding (a) how close they are to reaching their goal and (b) their level of confidence that things will continue to improve.

Goal achievement

- How will you know that you don't need to come here anymore?
- Who else will know?
- How convinced are you that you're on track now to getting what you want?
- How convinced are you that change will continue to happen?

Predicting what the future will look like helps clients with progress in the present. With practice it is also possible for practitioners to predict the number of sessions, as we shall see in the chapter on care aims. An example of this is Sandra, the lady with a stammer mentioned earlier (p. 42) who experiences pre-session change.

In the first session Sandra completes the WASSP assessment (Wright and Ayre, 2000). Although her stammer is hardly noticeable, you can see from the horizontal lines marked 1 in the summary profile that she considers her communication to be a major problem before therapy (Figure 3.1). However, using the miracle question she is able to identify possible solutions quite easily. It is agreed that Sandra will get in contact with the department when she wants another appointment.

After several months the therapist sends a letter enquiring whether Sandra wants any further input, and that unless she hears anything to the contrary she will presume that therapy is no longer needed. Sandra rings to make an appointment, and when they meet she tells the therapist that she was made redundant not long after her first session. She gives a long list of strategies and helpful activities she has been doing when asked how she has coped with this situation. The therapist feels that it would be useful to repeat the WASSP assessment, and when this is done they both look at how the results (Time 2) compare to the first results (Time 1) made six months previously. In the discussion of the profile Sandra says 'It [the stammer] isn't stopping me at all from doing things.'

The practitioner knows that significant change can occur in only two sessions, and uses the outcome measure (WASSP Summary Profile) to highlight this. Sandra feels she does not need further therapy. 'Because of the steps taken to promote independence and a sense of responsibility by clients about their changing, there is no need for a formal processing of concluding therapy' (Walter and Peller, 1992). It may be this sense of independence that allows Sandra to continue without further assistance, despite more positive change still needed socially and in the workplace. The therapist does not unilaterally decide the end of therapy or base it on a 'good' outcome in an

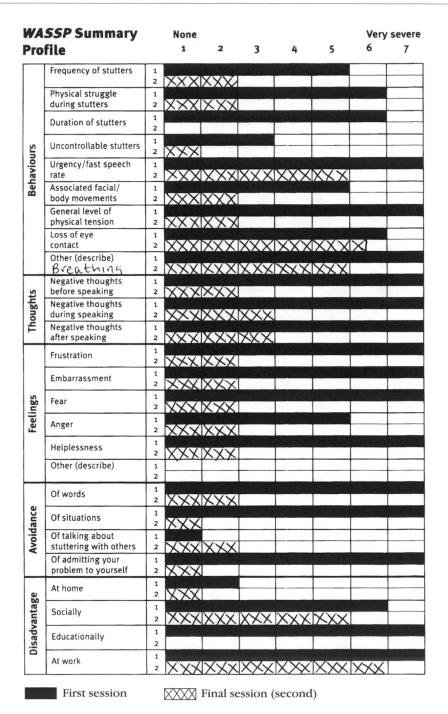

Figure 3.1 Sandra. Reproduced with permission from WASSP: Wright & Ayre Stuttering Self-Rating Profile, Louise Wright and Anne Ayre, Speechmark Publishing/ Winslow Press, Bicester, 2000.

assessment. SFBT encourages a collaborative approach. Because of this there does not need to be 'counselling' regarding the end of therapy.

Positive results from a formal assessment do not always help clients feel that they are managing communication effectively. Another client has residual speech and memory problems as a result of a transient ischaemic attack (TIA): 'Others tell me my speech is fine after the small stroke I've had, but I don't feel it is.' A dysarthria assessment is done which identifies minimal reduction in lip and tongue movement and some shallow breath support, but speech is 100 per cent intelligible. The results are shown to the client, but he remains unhappy. Another therapist is asked to assist with his case to see if SFBT can help. It turns out that it is the memory problems that are of real concern, and looking at how effectively he is coping with this area of his life appears to be the encouragement he needs.

Single session

Any client can feel their needs have been met with a single session, regardless of the complaint that causes them to look to a professional for help. To see if there are any common characteristics, it is easiest to look at case examples.

'I forget words and people's names. I forget why I'm on the phone. Today I got in the car and I had to drive round and round because I forgot how to get here.' This difficulty with memory, which like the previous client may be as a result of frequent TIAs, can result in a reduced capacity to process language. They are familiar clients in many speech and language therapy caseloads, but the reality of whether the therapist can make a difference with language is questionable. However, a single SFBT session can help clients realize that they are doing everything they can to make life manageable. This client who gets lost is more organized than he initially appears. For example, he has established a system for himself before leaving the house; he first thinks of the most important things he needs (keys, glasses, medicine), and he then thinks of the next category of importance (handkerchief), followed by the next (pencil, book). He has a list for key opening remarks for the telephone (if he forgets why he is on the phone). The therapist compliments him on his categorization skills and ability to prioritize, and encourages him to do more of the same.

Marking themselves on a scale can help clients realize that they are already well on their way to finding solutions to their problem. Mohammed has had a stroke two months previously and is still concerned about his speech, which he places at 7.5 on a scale. He also puts himself at 7.5 in terms of how confident he is that his speech will continue to improve. One session is sufficient for him to realize that 'Sometimes I can speak normally' and to identify how he can do this more often.

Marta has difficulties with her voice which is related to stress and anxiety. She is encouraged to think of what the future would look like if 'a little bit of magic happened' and she is able to be more relaxed. A long list of activities emerge which range from taking a bath and cleaning the flat to seeing her friends. She feels she can do these things without further assistance: 'In my life I have everything to do myself. I am determined. I think I alright. I thank you for listening to me.'

Another client also finds thinking about the preferred future is the trigger that gets him going. He has come to discuss his stammer, but he chooses to talk about goals that are quite unrelated to his speech. 'I will say hello to my mother in the morning and have a shave to please her.' He does not feel the need to take up the offer of a further appointment.

Key point

- The single session does not appear to be related to whether clients think they will be 'cured'. Clients with Parkinson's disease have come for a single session; despite the multiplicity of problems that can occur with this disease it is not inevitable that these clients will want to stay on the caseload.

Clients are always told that they are welcome to contact the department again themselves (if they feel their communication deteriorates) or that they can be re-referred via the doctor, nurse or consultant (if there are concerns with their swallowing).

Single sessions are not viewed as a fluke. It appears that SFBT techniques can enable clients to feel they do not have to rely on a large number of professionals unless a specific need arises. Giving clients the choice as to whether they want to be seen or not is dealing with them in a more respectful, as well as an ultimately more effective, way.

Self determination

Surely many of our needy clients will choose therapy that goes on as long as possible rather than brief therapy, if given the choice? This is not borne out by our experience at the Chelsea and Westminster Hospital or by studies on the average number of SFBT sessions in other locations (see Chapter 8). The study on adolescents with learning difficulties (Thompson and Littrell, 1998) is based on two counselling sessions and two follow-up interviews which do not include counselling. Comments on the outcome include 'It was fun and helpful', 'It was short and to the point', and 'He gave me confidence.'

A single-session case example of an 18-year-old boy with mild learning difficulties may illustrate how SFBT can help encourage clients' ability to make choices, and meet some of their need for increased confidence. Chris is concerned about the quality of his voice and that he cannot articulate the thoughts in his head. 'I need more confident speech. I'm doing well for myself. I want to prove to people that they're wrong – I *can* do it'. When asked the miracle question this is his reply:

Chris:	I wouldn't be asking my sister where things are all the time. I'd be talking less and speaking more slowly. I would leave [for work] on time and not leave anything behind.
Therapist:	What would other people notice you doing differently?
Chris:	I'd be more comfortable with my sister. She'd notice that I was getting on with her. My Mum would see that she doesn't need to keep telling me things.
Therapist:	Anybody else notice anything different?
Chris:	My boss would see that I'm more organized on my desk and all the work is finished. I'd be listening more, and understanding questions people ask.

Chris is already at a number 6 and will settle for 9 in terms of how he is managing overall. He is at 8 regarding how confident he feels that things will continue to improve.

Therapist:	How will you know this session has been useful to you?
Chris:	When I leave now I'll be smiling. It's useful you telling me I'm confident and I'm doing something well.

Chris leaves the room telling himself that he is confident, not the therapist doing it for him. A follow-up appointment is made, but he does not attend as he is at college.

With respect to clinical and educational emphases, the recent past has witnessed dramatic growth in the development of interventions designed to teach individuals with developmental and learning disabilities to understand their own abilities and needs, set goals for themselves, solve problems, manage their own affairs, advocate for themselves, and create the necessary supports to facilitate their participation in these processes. (Ylvisaker, Jacobs and Feeney, 2003, p. 17)

> **Key point**
>
> ■ SFBT facilitates the training in awareness and choice making which is a critical part of work with those who suffer brain damage.

Damien, who suffered a traumatic brain injury, was unable to do the miracle question without assistance from his girlfriend as we have seen earlier (p. 51). However, looking at exceptions and using scales appears to be useful; he puts himself at 8 in terms of independence but says 'It will take time. I may never get back to how I was.' He has problems with memory ('I've lost seven mobile phones in the last ten months'), fatigue, reduced comprehension and poor carryover from the sessions. Neither the therapist nor the girlfriend feel that 8 is a realistic figure, but its importance is that it is a measure of where he feels he has come from, and his comment reveals that there is insight into how much further he will be able to go. Damien is seen for three sessions over a period of five weeks. He applies for an art course, gets out of the house more and plans to attend a group with other clients with TBI. These activities will be more use to him than extensive one to one therapy as a hospital outpatient. When asked how the sessions have been useful to him he replies: 'I've been able to talk about myself which I don't often do ... how I feel ... get things off my chest. I feel more confident.'

Ahmed, another client with TBI, sees his problems as talking too much, losing his turn, saying things out of context, having difficulty with his concentration and feeling that 'my tongue sometimes pronounces a word differently. My confidence is not like it used to be. At the moment even crossing the road is a big task.' The therapist works with the principle that it is more effective to begin therapy by identifying what is working for the individual in everyday routines (handicap/participation) rather than starting with work on impairments in communication. This alternative model proposed by Ylvisaker et al. (1999) reverses the hierarchy common in traditional cognitive retraining approaches in TBI rehabilitation, which were based on starting therapy with largely unsuccessful cognitive exercises (particularly with memory) in clinical settings. So that generalization occurs, new learning and the practice of skills need to take place as much as possible with 'real-world tasks' in everyday settings.

SFBT helps with work on real-world tasks. It uses clients' language to formulate goals and measure change. Furthermore, it can help with a critical component of rehabilitation for many people with TBI which is to 'reconstruct an organized and positive sense of personal identity' (Ylvisaker and Feeney, 2000). Ahmed is able to imagine a preferred future with the therapist, and concludes by saying:

Ahmed: I want to impress myself.
Therapist: Focus on one small step so that you can impress yourself.

He arrives at the next session having taken a bus on his own for the first time since his accident, and he identifies this as an important step. When asked how therapy has been useful to him he says:

Ahmed: This has helped me notice ... see what I need to do so I don't close in on myself at home.

Like Damien, Ahmed is not seen for a large number of sessions. More is not necessarily better, just as a thirty-minute session can be as useful as a one hour session, particularly for someone who has difficulty concentrating. The aim of therapy is not to remove all of Ahmed's problems, many of which are likely to remain. It is to help him notice small but significant solutions, and enable him to find the confidence to know when and where to ask for help.

Spacing sessions

SFBT is focused on what clients are noticing that works well in their lives and how this is being achieved. In order to facilitate this, and help them feel a growing sense of control over their lives, the interval between sessions is determined by the client. This is very different to traditional therapy models that plan one or more sessions regularly every week.

Usually the time between sessions is lengthened as clients become more confident in noticing solutions. If a homework task has been set, then clients need time to perceive a difference that is meaningful to them and see that change has come about through their own resources. This is a particularly useful concept when taking on clients who have become dependant on therapy. Insoo Kim Berg demonstrates her skills with such a client:

I'm really impressed by how it is clear to you what you need to do. You're really aware of what's good for you and what isn't.
My suggestion at this point is to say: 'Just do it!' You've learnt how to do things yourself and take steps ... Now when you have enough steps, ring, and come and tell x about them. You give yourself about six or seven weeks. You don't want to be told – you decide what those steps are. Good luck. (Ratner, 1999)

Another way of phrasing the end of this would be to say: 'When you're ready to take the next step, you can come and talk about what you're going to do.'

The following examples illustrate the different packages of care given to clients already mentioned. Other examples are given later in the book when dealing with multidisciplinary issues (which include clients whose therapists feel they need help with 'moving on').

*   Cecil has five sessions over four months when first seen. He re-refers himself two years later and has one session (when he notices an improvement in how he is coping with PD). Two years later he is seen once when admitted to hospital.
*   James is referred by a colleague for specific SFBT input to help with his level of frustration as a result of his stroke. He is seen for three sessions over a period of three weeks.
*   Andrew is referred five months after his stroke. He has one session, and arranges for the next session to be three months later. The final session is six months after this.

All three clients are encouraged to do what they feel is helpful to them and to give themselves time to notice differences in their lives. Practitioners can of course make suggestions (see end of Chapter 4). The timing of sessions does not always follow expectations: one client, despite significant problems with her speech and language after a stroke, does not want any help when she is discharged from hospital. She returns as an outpatient eight months later and is seen for two sessions.

Key points

■   Clients decide on the interval between sessions
■   Increased confidence tends to lengthen this time
■   Clients can decide when to start and end therapy

Creative thinking

SFBT does not claim to be unique in using many of the ideas discussed in this chapter. Influences of other nondirective therapy techniques can be seen both in the language used, and the way intervention is given as briefly as possible. What is suggested here is that SFBT promotes creative thinking as to how you offer assistance to your clients, and this may challenge some previously held beliefs or departmental procedures.

Practitioners in SFBT have offered screening appointments, phone counselling and walk-in clinics in order to help reduce waiting lists. Some invite clients, especially adolescents, to e-mail between sessions to keep them informed on the way things are going in their lives. These different forums appear to work principally because it is the clients who are doing the work; they are responding to specific questions about their solutions, they are imagining their preferred future and working with scales, and communication impairments do not necessarily stand in the way of this process.

Practitioners themselves need to believe that crises can be resolved briefly, and you will soon see evidence of this in your caseload. The following letter is from a man with a moderately severe stammer. After two sessions he has been obliged to move house and job suddenly, and is no longer able to attend therapy, so he writes a letter to the therapist: 'The effect [of moving] on my speech has been non-existent! The fluency and communication I have now are at the same level as when we last met. In the short space of time I spent with you I found your help and words and techniques very effective and professional, so many thanks for that. I think your outlook is one I will carry [*sic*] now, with little deviance.'

Key points

- Your clients are the experts on themselves
- SFBT practitioners help them to recognize this

Summary

This chapter has focused in more detail on some of the assumptions of SFBT. There is the belief that pre-session change is not unusual and that the practitioner will find the clients competences, even if some clients *appear* to be noncompliant. This is useful to bear in mind when reading clients referrals, along with the ability to look for the unexpected. Setting tasks for them to do at home also encourages clients to develop this ability. The SFBT approach encourages you to begin to manage your caseload differently by assuming there may be resolution within one session or a short number of sessions spaced over a period of time determined by the client. Because the language you use in the session is solution focused this will also be reflected in the reports you write on discharge.

Chapter 4
Kate's story: 'I've had enough!'

This first session has been given in its entirety for two reasons. First, when the therapist looked at the video recording, she realized there are a number of SFBT questions used which follow the first session 'format', and it is helpful to see them in context. (The exception to this is the miracle question; it is asked later in the session for clarification, as Kate has already begun to identify how life will be without the problem.) Second, there is a lot of complimenting and repetition by the therapist which forms part of the process of enabling Kate to see her situation in a different light. Those unfamiliar with SFBT may find this useful.

It is not a 'perfect' session, and although some of the feedback given is specific to people who stammer, the point to remember about SFBT is its universality of application. Whenever someone asks Steve de Shazer 'How do you use SFBT with x?' (*some diagnostic category goes in here*), he tends to ask them to role-play the person they are thinking of. That way they are able to realize that it is not about working with concepts but with people.

Kate, 22 years old, is referred by her doctor for help with her stammer, and is seen for three sessions. Each session lasts about 60 minutes.

On the first occasion Kate arrives with her mother, who is invited in to the session by the therapist and Kate. The therapist knows nothing about Kate other than she has just begun a course at college, has had some speech and language therapy (SLT) in the past, and that her speech continues to cause her some distress.

The first session

Problem-free talk/problem definition

Therapist:	You've been to this hospital before?
Kate:	No, I haven't. I first went to a speech therapist when I was about 7, and that was in the old children's hospital ... You see – I'm talking fine now, but it does ...

71

Mum: (*interrupts*) Telephone work – terrible ...

Kate: Telephone ... I just will not get on the phone. I won't even speak to my grandparents ... I haven't spoken to my grandparents for fear of stammering. Anything that goes wrong in my house I always get my partner to phone up. He's fed up of dealing with everything because basically I just will not get on the phone. I get very nervous when I go to meet new people, don't I? (*turning to Mum*) I mean, I really work myself up. I've been given some tablets by the doctor ... and I just started to do it then: 'err ... err ...' and I will start saying funny words like 'like', you know, just to try and get myself over it. And it's extremely embarrassing sometimes because I'm sure some people look at me and think, 'My God, what's the matter with her, she was fine a minute ago?' and suddenly I just ...

Mum: And also your colour as well. It just flushes red.

Kate: Yeah. I get extremely red and I do actually suffer from a lot of rashes, and I've been told it's probably related to this because I get myself so worked up.

Mum: Psoriasis ... she had it in her scalp at one point.

Kate: Yeah.

Mum: Well, I get eczema. So I think in my family we're all very scratchy people. We're always scratching something. But mine isn't related to nervousness or anything. Hers is. You can tell. You can see her colour change ...

Therapist: So if I see you get redder in this room ...

Kate: (*laughing*) It will probably be this hot jumper.

Therapist: Yes. It's hot in here. We can always turn the fan on. Bear that in mind. Okay ... that's briefly how you see your speaking. I mean ... initially ... from my point of view... it [the speaking] sounds wonderful but ...

Kate: It's not always like that though.

Therapist: I absolutely appreciate that if you feel it's ... that you're aware there are difficulties. That's the issue. Just to mention – with the 'like's and 'er's, we obviously all do that. I say them loads. It sounds perfectly normal. But the issue is what you feel about it so ...

Kate: And then ... yeah ... I can't speak now. It's just sometimes nothing will come out. And I'll be fighting it, and trying to breathe, and trying to breathe, and counting to 10 in my head. I feel I'm a bit of a freak to be honest. It's so embarrassing for me sometimes.

Therapist: I notice that you've been to some speech therapy in the past, from this letter I got from the GP.

Kate: Yeah.

Mum: Primary school it was.

Kate: When I was 7 I went. Because I was being picked on a little bit and I think that's what triggered it off. And then I went to state school for years and completely got over it. Then I actually went through a period of not working, didn't I? (*looking at Mum*) I think I got a little bit depressed or something. And that's what made it come back. Do you remember? ... I was on to the phone, crying and stuff. That's when the stammering started to come back.

Therapist: How was speech therapy helpful to you?

Kate:	Well. So far as I remember I drew a little picture. I don't remember going any more than once. Apparently I went twice.
Mum:	At least two or three times. I didn't go in the room. A little chat, literally that's all they did. And then at school I think they liaised a little bit but then you moved to another class.
Kate:	Yeah. It just completely went. I didn't even think about it.
Mum:	I mean this girl's danced. She got on stage in front of ... I mean she can happily do that! And then she has a problem picking the phone up.
Kate:	Yeah. That's exactly what I mean.
Mum:	I think the last few months she's been a lot better. She's just started a course.
Kate:	Yeah. I'm training to be a nursery school teacher. I mean the last thing I want to do is teach the children stuttering, 'cause it might come through. And also it gets quite hard for me at college sometimes, like in a couple of week's time I have to do a verbal presentation, and the thought of that is just really, really ...
Mum:	Maybe you could do it in rhyme...
Therapist:	So dance is the thing that you really like, is it?
Kate:	Yeah. Unfortunately I can't dance, through a disc prolapse. So I think that also didn't help with making me feel depressed and things, because I couldn't ... and ever since then I started to go a bit downhill.
Therapist:	What kind of dance was it?
Kate:	I used to do classical dancing. Ballet, things like that. Didn't look like this then. (laughing) That was a while ago now.
Therapist:	And where do you go to do nursery nursing?
Kate:	I go down the college in the evenings and work in a nursery during the day.
Therapist:	Which college?
Kate:	X . It's an excellent course. A very good course.

The therapist now decides to establish the goal of the session. Kate begins the session talking fast, with a lot of body movement (scratching her arms, fiddling with the neck of her jumper) but, as seen from this transcript, there are few overt signs of a stammer, other than when she alerts the listener that she is struggling with her words.

The therapist tries to acknowledge her difficulties, and at the same time give some reassurance that 'fillers' in speech, such as 'like' and 'er' are quite normal. She does not pursue Kate's line of thought regarding the possible causes of the stammer.

Although some time is spent on problem talk, as both Kate and her mother show a need to talk about this, there is also a lot of problem-free talk embedded in the conversation. The therapist could develop some of this further. It does not always have the preferred outcome; asking about the dancing reveals another problem (disc prolapse)!

Key points

*   How has therapy been helpful in the past?
*   What's Kate doing at the moment?
*   What does she like doing?

After giving a few factual details not related to speech, the therapist feels that
Kate is calmer, and able to focus on the goal for the session.

Goal for the session

Therapist:	So how do you think I might be helpful to you today?
Kate:	Give me some breathing techniques, or give me something to just get over this type of thing where I go 'can't speak, help, help!' and I start to panic. If there's any sort of breathing ... or some ...
Mum:	I would say medically as well you've always had problems with your glands and breathing. I mean she's very blocked now because she's got a cold. That's nearly all the time. I mean she's really bad at the moment, but all the time she's really sinusy, coughing or feeling hot and rashy. And it all ... with her breathing and the speech, it all really does get blocked. Sometimes you do actually phone me now and again ... I can't understand what she's saying on the telephone.
Kate:	Yeah. I just tend to rush it or I'll just end up crying basically.
Mum:	(*interrupts*) So I'm not sure that you'll get rid of all the sinusy problem anyway that you have.
Kate:	I don't know if that's related. I think it's just in my head with the stammer. I think I possibly make it worse by building myself up. By getting so nervous beforehand, and I'll just think, 'Oh God, I can't do it, I can't do it', rather than just forgetting about it. About this talking thing; because I'm constantly thinking about talking to other people, I'm so, like, worried about the stammering. If someone could do something and take away this phobia I have about speech, then I'll probably be fine.

Notice that Kate is able to clarify her own goals rather than have them given
to her by her mother. The therapist does not address the 'sinusy' issue. Nor
does she question whether it is possible that someone could do something
and 'take away this phobia'. Instead, she hopes to look at the times when
Kate is less problem focused, find out if she is aware of any exceptions, and
explore how the exceptions may have happened. It is especially important
to use the client's language here.

Exceptions

Therapist:	Tell me about the times when you *do* forget about it.
Kate:	When I'm at home with me fiancé I don't really tend to think about it, although sometimes I will be talking to him about something

	that's happened to me or whatever and I will start a little bit. And I'll go 'Oh God, I can't speak now' and he'll turn round and say 'Yes you can, go on', then I'm like... I'm doing it now
Mum:	(*interrupts*) See now ... she'll tell me every time. That's another thing she's started to do now.
Kate:	Yeah. I have to tell people ...
Mum:	... 'I'm stammering now'. No you're not! But it's a break in the conversation and she thinks 'I've just blown this stream of what I'm going to say therefore I'm stammering now.' But a lot of people do that every day.
Kate:	... because I tend to run out of breath. Because I try to get it all out so quickly that I go ... (*demonstrates deep breath*) . . . 'I can't say the next bit'.
Therapist:	What is it about being with your fiancé at home that means that you are able to 'get it out'?
Kate:	Because I'm in my own home. Because he knows that I suffer from this. He doesn't try to speak for me or anything else like that, he'll just turn round ... not basically even take a blind bit of notice to it. He'll just completely ignore it. I think possibly because I feel comfortable with him, I'm not scared of talking to him. I'm not worried of what he may think. Which you know ...
Mum:	Can I ask a question? Since she started in college in the evening ... (*turning to Kate*) How many is there now in the college?
Kate:	There's about 18 of us to a class.
Mum:	And is it like a classroom where she [the teacher] comes round and asks questions, or you put your hand up?
Kate:	Yeah.
Mum:	And are you doing that alright now?
Kate:	Yeah, sometimes but ...
Mum:	It's sometimes that you wish you could ask the question.
Kate:	Yeah, that's the problem because I'm sure sometimes people think I'm a bit dim or something 'cause I'm just too scared to talk, and I just sit there very quiet. I'm sure people think 'Oh gosh, she's really boring.' It's just I'm too scared of making a fool of myself I think.
Therapist:	Let's come back to that in a minute, because I think you're right, the college is a difficult situation ... I mean, groups are difficult, for all of us. We can all find groups, standing up, presentations, a difficult situation. To go back to you, at home with your fiancé ... You're saying that you know ... you're at home ... he obviously sounds lovely! He ignores ...
Kate:	He just completely ignores it. He doesn't make a big issue out of it.
Therapist:	Okay (*reading from notes*) ... that he doesn't try to speak for you. What is it that you're doing differently though, because you're right, he's doing all the right things, but what are *you* doing differently that means that you can *not* think about it ... talk normally ... all of that?
Kate:	Probably because I'm not thinking about this stammer when I talk to him, it's just when I talk to other people. You know, I get really ... it's always at the front of my mind when I talk with other people, but not with him.
Therapist:	So what are you doing instead?

Kate:	Just talking. Not thinking about the stammering.
Therapist:	You just talk.
Kate:	Yeah.
Therapist:	And you're feeling ...
Kate:	I feel fine then 'cause I just don't think about it. Just as soon as I step outside or if that phone rings, I say 'Ben!' (*fiancé's name*) and he says 'Can't you answer it?' and I won't. I just let it ring and ring, and it has actually caused us to fight sometimes. Because I will not answer the phone. I'll tell you something else that happens. He'll phone twice, put the phone down and then phone back so that I'll answer it.
Mum:	I had to do that the other day. Phone twice, leave it and then you ring me back.
Kate:	Yeah, so that I know it's certain people, because otherwise if someone just phones you about something else I just will not be able to speak to them.
Therapist:	Sorry to keep going back to that situation ... Really, the key to looking at all of this is not thinking that everything is out of your control. Well, you can't control the group in college, you can't stop the phone ringing. Environments where you *do* feel in control ... which is with your fiancé. There's something about that that enables you to be calm.
Kate:	Yeah, just to talk and not to worry about it.
Therapist:	And that's because *you* are the expert on how you talk. I see lots of people who come here and who have stammers but I'm not the expert; the expert is you, because you know better than anyone (your fiancé, your Mum, anybody), exactly what works for you. So to go back to that moment, just that one moment, say, where you 'just talk'; you *do* know.
Kate:	I know. I'm not even thinking about it.
Therapist:	So in terms of any secret cures, or breathing exercises ... Are you thinking about your breathing then?
Kate:	I think I'm probably more relaxed then. There have been times when I do actually stammer with him.
Therapist:	Sure. Absolutely. But the times when you're not stammering ... what do you think is happening with you breathing? Do you think it's ...?
Kate:	I'll talk very quickly and get it all out, and then I'll just relax a little bit, and then ...
Therapist:	Is that just with your fiancé?
Kate:	It's funny, sometimes I can talk fine, and I can meet someone new and can talk fine, but then suddenly something will happen ... I don't know what it is. I'll just not be able to say another word and I'll end up ...
Therapist:	Okay, with your fiancé you can sometimes talk fine. With other people you're saying you can, sometimes ...
Kate:	Sometimes. Yeah.
Therapist:	So that would be ... what ? Anybody? Even complete strangers?
Kate:	Sometimes. Yeah.
Therapist:	Who else? Who else can you talk fine with? Your Mum?
Kate:	Yeah.
Mum:	Your brother.

Kate:	Not with x – I talk funny. Yeah, it's funny that.
Mum:	Do you!
Therapist:	All the time, or sometimes?
Kate:	Most of the time. He's 13, and it tends to be a bit more embarrassing with him.
Therapist:	But would you say that's 100 per cent of the time or sometimes?
Kate:	I'd say with him that was about 70 per cent of the time. It's fine when I'm telling him off, and when I'm having an argument. It's just when I'm talking normally.
Therapist:	What do you think it is about telling him off that means that you can speak more fluently?
Kate:	It means that I'm in control of the situation and he does as I say! (*laughing*)
Mum:	He doesn't visit often, you can tell!
Therapist:	So it sounds like it's a little bit the feeling of being in control.
Kate:	Yeah. I think it's all about control, with me. I have to feel comfortable and safe in a situation before I can talk normally.
Therapist:	Again, we all have a bit of that, don't we? We all feel comfortable at home. Hopefully, we feel comfortable with Mum, Dad ... so things tend to work well in that situation.

During this section the therapist feels Kate is increasingly able to focus on the exceptions. She mentions that talking with the fiancé is easier. She is then able to recognize that sometimes she is able to talk to strangers, even though previously she has said 'new people' are difficult.

Notice how the therapist keeps bringing the conversation back to the times when Kate feels things are working better for her. She listens to the problem talk, but brings Kate back to being solution focused by saying 'Let's come back to that in a minute' or 'Sorry to keep going back to that situation.' The aim is (a) to get more details of the times when the preferred future is already happening, and (b) for Kate to experience the satisfaction of knowing that parts of her life already exist without the problem.

She can feel an expert and know for herself what works; she is able to say '*I know*', which is very empowering. The therapist is constantly feeding back to her and using her words; 'talk fine' and 'comfortable' appear key. Notice how the therapist does not restrict language to the 'problem', and is using the phrase 'talk fine' without necessarily clarifying whether this means talking with, or without, a stammer. What is important is that Kate feels comfortable with her speech.

Kate says she sometimes feels she's 'a freak'. The therapist is normalizing some of the examples by pointing out that they can be stressful for everyone, but it is probably the process of going over the exceptions in detail that Kate is able to absorb the calming effect and be able to find the reassurance for herself, which is infinitely more valuable. Her mother appears to be listening more than at the beginning of the session.

> **Key points**
>
> ■   When does Kate forget about her stammer?
> ■   What's helpful about being with her fiancé?
> ■   What's she doing then?
> ■   When are the other times she can 'talk fine'?

The therapist feels that getting some precise measure of where Kate is, and where she wants to get to, will be useful now.

Scales

Therapist:	(*getting pen and paper for Kate*) Okay … let's just try …
Mum:	She's drawing a picture!
Therapist:	No. It's just a line. I want to look at this line … (*drawing*), and you'll notice that here we've got a 0, and up here we've got a 10. Now … 0 is when things are at their worse, when maybe stammering is quite bad, and 10 is when things are pretty good. Where would you say you are now?
Kate:	Right now?
Therapist:	Now. Generally. Where would you say you are between 0, being really, really bad, and 10 being …?
Kate:	About 5. Shall I make a mark? Somewhere in the middle (*marks line*).
Mum:	And her rash is coming up! (*pulling at the neck of Kate's jumper*)
Kate:	(*ignores Mum*) Yeah, because I'm fine sometimes, and sometimes I'm terrible so …
Therapist:	Nobody says you're stuck at 5, because we all fluctuate. We have days when we're right down in the dumps and low, and other days when things are just great. Aiming for the 10?
Kate:	Oh God yeah! I just want to talk normally. That's all I want to do.
Therapist:	(*drawing*) So … in *this* line, 0 is that you aren't confident at all that things get better and improve, and 10 is that you are confident that things can get back to normal. Where would you say you are now?
Kate:	What about things getting better? (*starts crying*) I would say about 3, because I don't feel things can be any better (*marks paper*).
Therapist:	Let's just go back to this [other] line. Now, you've given me a 5, and you've already told me about situations which are difficult, like the telephone. The telephone is well known to be a difficult thing for loads of people. I loathe the telephone, and I read in a book somewhere that if you stood up while talking on the phone it helped confidence! If at the moment you're not able to talk on the phone, then that's quite tough for you. How have you managed to be at 5? You could have told me you were stuck at 2 or 3.
Kate:	I think probably just because I tend not to answer the phone ever, and I tend not to shop by myself or ever ask for anything. I won't ask the cab driver to take me anywhere. I'll always write it down on a piece of paper and say 'Can you take me there please?' I'll

	even laugh and joke with them, but it's just the thing that ... you know, just giving people information ... I'm scared. So I will actually write even my own home address on it. I've got so many little secret ways of doing things so that I don't have to speak it.
Therapist:	But that's you managing to get out and about. It's not as if you're sitting at home never going out and never seeing anybody. You're not doing that. You haven't told me that's what you're doing. You're saying 'I have lots of strategies' ...
Kate:	Yeah I do, honestly, which people would laugh at ... People must think I'm mad.
Therapist:	But those are the strategies that are useful to you. Nobody would say they are wrong. They are useful to you.
Kate:	Yeah. They help me.
Therapist:	So what else are you doing to stay at that number 5? Because you're obviously doing quite a lot to get out and about.
Kate:	I've started going to college. I'm working at the nursery. I am trying to get over it. I've basically now had enough of it, and it's just like a constant everyday thing, but I think I make it worse by thinking about it. It's always, always on my mind. I'll tell you something which was really funny. A few weeks ago we went to the doctor, didn't we (*to Mum*), and he gave me these tablets. He said they would calm me down, bring down my blood pressure and things.
Mum:	Almost like anti-depressants, weren't they?
Kate:	No, no, no. They're for blood pressure and things. You don't get all panicky because, you know, I was about to start college – do you remember? – and I'd taken two beforehand. Well, you know, because I'd taken these two tablets, in my head I could suddenly get rid of the stammer for that whole evening. I was fine. I was laughing [although] I was still nervous. Because I'd taken these tablets, I'd almost fooled myself into thinking that this had got rid of it. I was picked up by my boyfriend afterwards, and I was saying the doctor's given me these tablets and they're fantastic. After all that it's a one-off, but it's funny that sometimes I can actually fool myself. That's why I think that half of it's in my head. If I could just get rid of that.
Therapist:	There does seem to be something about that ... with a stammer ... that people don't know exactly what causes it. How much is the psychological ... and it's like a snowball, once something doesn't work ...
Kate:	Yeah, once you do it ...
Therapist:	... and that's perfectly valid and real. There are lots of theories on it and ideas as to why and how it happens. What we *do* know at the moment is that there is no cure. No magic cure.
Kate:	I know.
Therapist:	What's impressed me is that you haven't come here today and said 'give me the cure'. You're very real. You know exactly what you're doing, when you're doing it, which is impressive. You've probably got a greater awareness of what you're doing than a lot of other people. There can be positive things about stammering. People do spend a lot of time looking at themselves and saying 'why am I

	doing this?' and they tend to know themselves pretty well. It sounds like you've been quite ingenious with yourself, thinking of these strategies, and you're showing a lot of imagination and resourcefulness to be able to get out and do things ... because you also sound like a very determined person. Would you say that's right?
Mum:	Scorpio! Yes!
Therapist:	I mean that's coming across very strongly. You're very determined, resourceful ... you're not letting this get in the way of things because even though you're saying it's hard ... you've just started college. That's a big step! You're also working. You've got a relationship that's obviously working well. It's pretty impressive actually. I think you're also aware that the tablets the GP gave you, although they might have made you feel better for a while ... that if they stop working, then what do you do?
	The point you've reached now [is] where you've said ... 'I want to be doing this myself, then if it's under my control and I know what I'm doing, it's not that someone can take it away from me. That's great – I've got it! And even though sometimes it might still work less well than at other times, I know what I'm doing and I'm in control.' That can be the problem with some of the courses people who stammer go on. They come away, they're talking really well, and three months later ...
Kate:	... it's not so good any more.
Therapist:	It's not to say I don't think courses aren't helpful. They are. But what are you holding on to at the end of the day? You need to see for yourself all the things that you're doing because when you start listing, at number 5, all the things that you're doing (*writes under Kate's 5*), which is: going to college, working ... What else are you doing? Doing any other ...?
Mum:	She's got a membership for the gym. Pilates ...
Kate:	Yeah. Just started at the gym.
Therapist:	(*writes*) Going to the gym.
Kate:	That's about it really, isn't it?
Mum:	You're managing a household, aren't you, with your fiancé? You know, cooking, and all that housewifely things.
Therapist:	So you've got your own place.
Mum:	She doesn't have her Mum doing everything. She's doing her own thing.
Therapist:	(*writes*) Running a home. That in itself ...
Kate:	Yes, but I just want to be able to talk normally, and not be worried.
Mum:	Yes, but you need to look at all the good things that she's doing because I think she tends to think negative quite a lot. 'Oh, I can't do that' or 'I've told people I can't do that so it's acceptable', but it isn't acceptable.
Therapist:	I think it's about you being able to see for yourself, because it's all very well me and your Mum admiring the energy you have ... and that you're obviously very capable and determined, as I said. You need to see it for yourself.
Kate:	I just wish I could talk and not have to worry.

Therapist:	The talking doesn't seem to be getting in the way of you managing your life. Sometimes we need to step back and notice we are doing an awful lot of things, because people who stammer sometimes use it as a safe thing to hold on to, because it's quite a nice excuse ... which is fine! Use that stammer as well if you want to. But the fact is that it hasn't stopped you from doing all these things. And my next thing would be to say, okay, let's think about one step up at 5.5/6. How would number 6 be different to number 5?
Kate:	Number 6 would be being able to talk on the phone I think. Or just being able to answer the phone.
Therapist:	With the phone ... Does that feel like a big step? (*Kate nods*) Yeah? Not a six then?
Kate:	Number 6 7 8 9 10!
Therapist:	Where would we put it then?
Kate:	9 or 10.
Therapist:	So we're going to put the telephone up here for a minute (*writes 'telephone' under Kate's 9/10*). You have your goals, but you're thinking 'Yeah, the telephone ... I'm working on that.' You're working on that. But 'how will I know things have got just a little bit better?' That's the key. We're going to start noticing a number 6. [Things] that you're doing now.
Kate:	I don't know ... I don't know.
Therapist:	Just something ... that would help you feel 'this feels a bit more comfortable for me, a bit more under my control'.
Kate:	I think ... there's so many things, but then there's really not.
Mum:	You may think there's nothing really. Today we got on a bus and we were chatting. That was fine. Then we got lost. So we grabbed a cab, and she asked me to tell him where we're going. She asked me to tell him, instead of her doing it.
Kate:	Yeah. Something like that. If I could just ...
Mum:	... open the door and say x, or your address.
Kate:	Yeah, possibly my own address
Therapist:	You'll have to be catching a lot of cabs in the next week or so! An expensive exercise! (*all laughing*)
Mum:	She's impatient. She doesn't like waiting for buses.
Therapist:	So you're impatient as well!
Kate:	Yeah. I want to talk *now*!
Therapist:	You *are* talking now! (*laughing*) It *is* a difficult thing to break things down a bit, because it's quite hard thinking that way. So some of the questions that I'm asking ... I know you might need time. It might be just one thing that would make a difference, and help you feel you were moving on a bit.
Kate:	I really don't know. I feel I just have this thing about the telephone ... the telephone ... the telephone.
Therapist:	I know. The telephone We haven't got rid of it. It's up there (*pointing to line*).
Kate:	Talking to people and not being scared of talking to people ... even friends of mine.
Therapist:	Okay. Let's think of it another way. Think about last week or the last couple of weeks. Maybe you've already been at a number 6,

	because we shift around, don't we? Last week when there was a moment with your friends and you felt 'Oooh, this feels really good'? A good day, evening ... Can you think of a time that was a particularly good moment?
Kate:	(*turning to Mum*) When you, me and x went out to dinner that night? Two Saturdays ago. We were all sitting together and chatting. (I don't drink, it makes me feel ill.) We were having a laugh altogether. I didn't stammer at all that night, did I?
Mum:	No one would ever notice. I certainly didn't.
Therapist:	So that was a number 6. Probably more than a 6?
Kate:	Yeah. Probably a 6 or 7.
Therapist:	So. The point is that you sort of already know what it feels like. It's not about me teaching you. You kind of already know. It's that you want to do more of that.
Kate:	Yeah I do. All the time.
Therapist:	What was it that you were doing that night? Okay, so it was a nice environment [but] there were things that you were doing that meant that you were ... free. Not drinking – you weren't even doing that. You were completely in control. How did you manage that?
Kate:	I think probably I was just sitting with family, and we were all just having a nice time. Other people were talking as well. I didn't have people staring at me and looking at me while I'm talking. I tend to ... if I'm talking with just one person and that person is just listening to me, that's when I panic I think. If it's a whole group of people all talking together and people listening to other people ... but it's just when I have someone staring at me I think 'Oh, I can't do this.' I think that sort of group thing; talking about the same subjects and putting our ideas ... Like, I'm going to college tonight. We're put into groups; then I'm fine. It's just if afterwards they have to have someone read things out. I'm dammed if I'm the one that's going to do it. No way!
Therapist:	What's interesting is that you've just said something which is actually unusual, in that often people tell me 'One to one is fine, it's in groups that I can't talk.'
Kate:	No, it's one to one, when someone's just looking at me.
Therapist:	Often people say groups are more difficult because conversation is fast and people are looking at you; because you say something, and *everybody* turns ...
Kate:	No, that's fine.
Therapist:	Do you see how what works for one person ...? You're the one that's important here. You're the one that's saying exactly ...
Kate:	Yeah. I feel much more comfortable cause we're all putting things in, and I can tend to hide this stammer then. You know, if there's a lot of people there I can get myself over it then. It's when I'm with the one person I just start freaking out a bit.
Therapist:	So in the group its something about you being able to say and feel what ...?
Kate:	... feel quite confident I suppose. I mean people do tend to laugh and that, you know, because I will actually tend to crack a joke

	here and there. I'm that sort of a person. Just to try to hide this stammer I think I become a bit more …
Therapist:	Well, you might be cracking jokes just because …
Kate:	(*interrupts*) No. I think part of it is this whole front.
Therapist:	Maybe that's part of it, but the other part is that you make people laugh. Great!
Kate:	Yeah.
Therapist:	You're a lively person. You're good news in a group because you can keep people entertained.
Kate:	Yeah, [I] certainly put down plenty of ideas and stuff. I mean, we have quite a lot of foreign girls in my group, so because of course I speak good English and write good English, I'm always the one who ends up with about four foreign girls asking me questions throughout the class: 'How do you spell that?' 'How do you …?' So that sort of thing I'm fine with. So that's when I feel more confident possibly because they need my help more then. I don't know. Maybe I just have this big ego trip.
Therapist:	You're using you're resources, because what you keep underlying is that it sounds like you *are* a confident person. I mean …
Kate:	Oh yes, really I am!
Therapist:	… you're able to talk in these groups, you're able to help those who need the help. You're going to go into a profession which is again helping people: kids.
Kate:	Of course.
Therapist:	In fact, you're already working in that. So you're using your resources really well. You're actually, it sounds like … you're more confident than you yourself realize. The thing is, what happens is that we don't notice it. We don't notice the times when things are working well. We notice the times …
Kate:	… yeah, the things that are really bad. Things are magnified.
Therapist:	So this is about you noticing a little bit more, as we're doing now. All the times you're getting on with life. You have your moments when you're not so good, but it's not stopping you from having a life, in fact.

Scaling questions appear to have been helpful to Kate. She is beginning to differentiate between dealing with what feels like a big issue for her (the telephone), and those areas of her life where the preferred future is already happening. The therapist could have chosen to use a specific scale to determine, for example, steps towards dealing with the issue of groups better: 0 could represent being in a family group which she can manage, and 10 is making a presentation in front of a group. But when she becomes tearful (looking at confidence level), the therapist decides to shift to some 'coping questions' and to spend time summarizing some of the positive points that have come up in the session.

Other options might have been exploring Kate's comment that things were fine for many years when at school. How did she manage that? It would also be interesting to ask some 'relationship questions': 'What would Mum notice you doing differently when you're at number 6?' 'What will she be doing differently?' Notice that Mum is trying to work with Kate on the scales, and she is able to recognize that her daughter is managing household things.

It can feel hard work striking the balance between shifting gear, when someone says 'I don't know', and asking the question again in a slightly different way. Rephrasing the question appears to work, when trying to elicit what a number 6 looks like. Watching the video, you can see Kate's response is immediate. You need to 'hang in there' and be aware that if a client is very problem focused, then noticing and thinking about solutions that may already exist can be difficult. The therapist has the advantage in that she knows the telephone is a common area of complaint (for anyone with a communication impairment), and that it is often improvement in another area that will increase confidence overall.

Key points

- On a scale, where is Kate now?
- Where does she want to be?
- How confident is she that things will improve?
- How has she managed to be at 5?
- Compliments
- How will she know she's reached 6?
- When have things been at a 6 in the last couple of weeks?

It seems a good point to ask Kate for more information about what life looks like without the problem: the therapist uses the miracle question to see if she can give as detailed a picture as possible of her 'number 10'. Interestingly, Kate has already commented on how she took two tablets and she 'got rid of' her stammer for an entire evening, and the therapist could pursue this theme of a 'magic pill'. What is important is that Kate feels the experience can be repeated and that it is not 'a one-off'.

Preferred future

Therapist:	Let's just try one other thing … and this is maybe going to sound a bit peculiar, but there's a reason behind it. I want you to imagine that after leaving here today … you going back to work now?
Kate:	No, no. Going home to study.
Therapist:	So, you're at home, and then … have supper …
Kate:	Then I'm at college later on this evening.
Mum:	It's her birthday today as well!
Kate:	I'm 23! I'm not happy at all!

Mum:	She said 'it doesn't feel like my birthday. I've got to go to college, and then I'm seeing the SLT!'
Therapist:	I saw it [the date] yesterday – I meant to say. Happy Birthday! Okay. So you're going to be celebrating a bit, maybe, tonight.
Kate:	I think I'll be too tired by the time I've finished.
Mum:	She's on antibiotics at the moment so I don't think she should be doing anything.
Kate:	I don't know … I might go for some dinner later.
Therapist:	Well. Okay. You're going to have a good day … the time comes to go to bed. You go to bed, and while you're asleep this miracle happens …
Kate:	Please! God! (*smiling*)
Therapist:	… and the miracle is that what brought you here today… some of the things that you've been mentioning, go … the problems go away. The thing is that tomorrow morning, you wake up, and you were asleep while this miracle was happening. So how do you know, when you wake up – tomorrow morning – that this miracle has happened? I want you to tell me what's the first thing that happens that tells you … 'Hey, this is amazing; this feels really different, this morning, than yesterday or the day before! Something really big has happened.' What are you doing that's different?
Kate:	The phone's ringing and I'm answering it and making phone calls myself to my friends, who must think I'm extremely rude because I never ever phone them back.
Therapist:	So you open your eyes and that's the first thing that happens?
Kate:	And the phone's ringing and it wakes me up and I rush over to the phone! (*laughing*)
Therapist:	Okay (*writing*). What else then?
Kate:	Um … when I go out with my friends, we're all sitting round and I don't at one point go 'err … err …', or feeling that feeling that I get.
Therapist:	But let's just … hang on a minute … you're doing an awful lot in the first five minutes! I'm trying to imagine the first few things that tell you … they might be really little things … that make you think 'Hey, something's different.'
Kate:	Nothing else apart from that. I honestly don't think anything else would actually make me realize, unless …
Therapist:	What would Ben notice?
Kate:	That I'm answering the phone.
Therapist:	What else would he notice? What would he notice you doing that was different?
Kate:	I don't know. Talking normally to him without any little blips or anything like that.
Therapist:	Would he notice that do you think?
Kate:	Yes. I think he would, especially when I'm chatting away to him. Yeah.
Therapist:	What else would he notice? I mean, it might be nothing to do with the talking. It might be something else.
Kate:	No rashes. No red blotches.
Therapist:	What else would he notice you doing differently?
Kate:	I don't know. I don't think there is anything else. (*silence*)
Therapist:	I know it's a funny question. It's a question …

Kate:	(*interrupts*) It's a hard question!
Therapist:	... that you can go away and think about. And obviously I'm not saying to you that I can make a miracle but it's a very useful thing to think about, because what you're sort of saying to me is that, well, things would be ...
Kate:	... would be the same as they are!
Therapist:	So what does that say to you then?
Kate:	That it's probably... all this is just me making things ...
Mum:	You're not making things up.
Therapist:	Not at all, no! But what else might it say to you?
Kate:	That I'm actually coping with it quite well and that, that my whole life doesn't actually revolve around this stammer! Yeah.
Therapist:	I couldn't put it in better words.
Mum:	Yeah.

The miracle question is best asked deliberately and dramatically; it is introduced as unusual or strange, and frequent pauses enables clients to process what is being said. Clients often give an answer that does not include well-formed goals, so it is then the task of the therapist to use follow-up questions. Kate is asked what her fiancé would notice that was different about her, to encourage her to describe possibilities in interactional terms. Later, the therapist introduces the idea that there may be one part of her miracle that would be easiest for her to do the next morning, so as to invite her to think about which possibilities are most realistic.

Future-directed words are used: 'What *are you doing* that's different?' 'What *would* Ben notice?' When clients say 'I don't know' try waiting a little longer in silence, as if you did not hear, as this can be taken as another cue to think harder and come up with a more complete answer. Who, what, when, where, and how questions can be asked to see if there are any indications that the miracle is already happening.

Key point

- After exploring the preferred future and being asked the question, 'What does that say to you?', Kate is able to acknowledge for herself that she is coping quite well and that her whole life doesn't revolve around her stammer.

Time is running short, so the therapist decides to give some session-ending feedback in order to organize and highlight

> the aspects of information that might be useful to clients as they strive to build solutions ... Compliments affirm what is important to the client ... [and] clients successes, and the strengths these successes suggest. (De Jong and Berg, 2002)

Feedback

Therapist: It's not to say that I don't absolutely recognize that you do spend time thinking about it [the stammer], but do you see how sometimes just stepping back ...? Suddenly people say, 'Well, you know x might notice a few umms and ahhs, sure, but ...'

Kate: (*interrupts*) Apart from that I'm not really that different a person, other than the fact that...

Therapist: Because there can be other people, in answer to that [miracle] question, who will list a lot of things ... and again, you can say, 'What *one* thing can you be doing now?' because it's about the things maybe that they're not doing, that's the issue for them. That maybe the stammer really is stopping them doing a whole lot of stuff. But in your case it sort of doesn't sound like that.

Kate: No.

Therapist: And it's about you being able to see that for yourself, really see that for yourself, because once you do that you'll start noticing the days and the weeks are okay ... and even with the telephone thing (that's you're goal, sure) you're thinking, 'I'm going to think about the 6 and 7, I'm not thinking about the 9/10 which is maybe the miracle thing.' And if you want to come back and see me again... and you say, 'I *did* notice something; I stood up in front of that group at college and that was alright'... actually, that sounds like a big one! (*all laughing*)

Kate: Yeah!

Therapist: You might come back with even just one thing, however small, and say 'that was a step for me' and the fact [is] that you noticed it yourself, and you didn't have somebody else saying 'Hey, you're doing fine'. Because you've got all these wonderful skills and resources, and it does sound like you're quite a confident person: you're very determined, you've done a hell of a lot of things in quite a short period of time. You've come here, and as you've said before: 'I've had enough!'

Kate: Yeah. I've had enough!

Therapist: Even just saying that is quite an empowering thing, isn't it? Sometimes stammers are useful, as I said, and you kind of live alongside it ...

Kate: For me it's not.

Therapist: Maybe you're just saying 'No, I've had enough of this'. And *you* said that!

Kate: Yeah. It's starting to get me down now.

Therapist: And it's how you're now going to put that to one side. It's how you're going to do that. It's not necessarily even going to be doing specific techniques, that you *have* to do. I mean, you'll notice I've given you no ...

Kate: I'm rather disappointed, actually! (*laughing*)

Therapist: Because, sure, you could say you've got to take a deep breath ... but how often do we do that ...? How useful is that really to you? It's maybe more useful for you to say, 'Well, let's look at the times when it's not an issue.'

Kate: When you *are* fine.

Therapist:	'What am I doing now? I'm comfortable, I'm relaxed.' Sure, the breathing probably is controlled, but that's on automatic. That's what you want.
Kate:	Yeah, That's exactly what I want.
Therapist:	And it's not a coincidence that when you were doing all these things, when you really have to be focused on something, that the talking thing actually wasn't an issue.
Kate:	Yeah. Never ever.
Therapist:	And it's about you being able to feel that. It's really sort of as simple as that. It's quite an empowering thing when you're able to do that, to notice when things work well, and seeing that you've already got the solutions. So if I just ask you one more question. Again, it might sound funny. At the beginning of the session you said to me ... when I asked you how I could be helpful to you ... (*reading*) 'If someone could *do* something', 'I just want to speak normally' um ... How do you think this session has been useful to you in terms of either sort of feeling some of that, and/or feeling you are a bit more in control?
Kate:	I think possibly just talking about these things that you put down, and having that scale where I can actually *see* I am, most of the time, at a 5. I'm not actually spending my whole life stammering, which is what it feels like. I'm not always, always, always stammering. And I'm not one of those people that go 'err ... err ... err ...', which is what I used to do – when I was 7 I used to do that – and go 'ss ... ss ... ss', and things like that. I don't do that any more. So I'm not spending my whole life stammering, which I did actually forget about, and it doesn't actually feel like such a big ... you know.
Therapist:	So when you walk out of this door now, what do you think you'll be doing differently?
Kate:	Just trying ... just trying to act like I act all the time when I'm talking normally. Just trying to feel that feeling, and not being preoccupied with this.
Therapist:	You know when it does feel right. I mean, you've been there.
Kate:	Oh yeah. And I'm actually there now, when I'm talking to you now, so it's not like it's always, always there. And I think if I try not to be so scared of when it *does* happen and just ... I think I just always fear ... and I shouldn't, because it's not happening at that time, so I shouldn't worry about it 'til it does.
Therapist:	I mean, sure, there are going to be situations that *are* scary situations for all of us, but because you know what to do and how to do it, you can say: 'That's okay; I know how to get back to the 5. And I'm thinking about the 6 and 7 now.'
Kate:	Yeah. Cool! (*big smile/thumbs up at the camera*)
Therapist:	Would you like to come back again?
Kate:	Yeah. Yeah.
Therapist:	Okay. You're going to have homework then!
Kate:	Okay then. More to add!
Therapist:	The homework is for you to come back and tell me the times you've been at a 6 and 7.

Kate:	So I have to list them as I'm doing them?
Therapist:	As you like, I don't mind. You can list them, you can give me just one. I don't mind.
Kate:	Okay. That's easy enough! (*looking at Mum/laughing*) I wish it was all like that!
Therapist:	Okay.
Kate:	Thank you very much.
Therapist:	So. You need a bit of time for that. When would you like to ...?
Mum:	Before you go away.
Kate:	Yeah. I'm going away to the Caribbean for Xmas ... So no, probably after I've come away because I think I'll probably have more to tell you ... because I've been away on holiday. Lots of 6s and 7s, won't I?
Therapist:	It's also about in everyday life. I mean I'm absolutely sure you'll be at a 9 or 10 after that! It's about not just thinking I have to be on holiday to get there. The everyday, as well.
Kate:	Okay, shall we say before I go?
	(*next appointment arranged for one month later*)
Therapist:	(*to Mum*) I hope it was useful for you, coming.
Mum:	Oh it was. I go with her to the doctors. I know how she feels so ...
Kate:	Because I tend to cry, you see.
Mum:	I don't mind if they say 'sit outside'. It's just me being here. The interview at college: I said 'I hope you don't mind!' and they said 'No, it's lovely to have a mother along.' I thought 'Oh, I'm not sure ...'
Kate:	Because I was quite scared of talking. She does tend to say a few words, and then I can.
Mum:	Otherwise she'll remain silent if I don't ... if I'm not. But I don't want to be a prop.
Therapist:	I'm sure, as you say, your presence is really useful.
Kate:	It just helps me relax a bit.
Mum:	If you haven't got anybody around ... just to go there is terrifying.
Therapist:	Especially the first time. Next time, you're welcome to come or not, it's up to you. (*turning to Kate*)
Kate:	I think I can manage it by myself! (*laughing*)
	(*all stand up/walk to door*)
Mum:	There you go ... it's another goal: 'I didn't ask my Mum to come down!' There's another thing: she rang me yesterday – she's not very well at all – and she said, 'I can't go into college. I feel terrible.' And I'm out with my boss and another colleague having lunch, and she says 'Please, please ... ring'. So she's rung me to say can I ring college, and I said I can't, and then I got a phone call later on saying, 'It's alright, I managed to do it!'
Kate:	Because she had an answer phone, so I could blurt it out really quickly: 'Hello, I'm not very well at all, but I shall be in on Thursday'. I'm just petrified of being asked questions.
Mum:	That was actually a feat for you to even think 'I've got to do that.'
Kate:	The reason why I did it is because I thought 'I'm going to the speech therapist tomorrow, I might as well start now!'
Therapist:	I'm not surprised by what you say. This whole way of working ... called Solution Focused Brief Therapy ... they find that before

people come to therapy, they start getting better. Again, it's back to ...
you're doing the work, not me. I can say to people, 'That doesn't
surprise me at all because you already know ...' It's such a positive,
empowering thing. You're off, even before you arrive here!
(*Kate and Mum leave room*)

There are frequent 'magic moments' in SFBT. For the therapist, the moment
when Kate smiles and puts her thumbs up at the camera is one of those.
There is a marked difference between the start of the session when Kate is
fidgety, anxious and crying and the end, when she is sitting calmly, smiling
and talking more slowly.

The therapist lets the camera run as they go to the door to leave and it
captures the throwaway comment from Mum regarding pre-session change.
It also shows that Mum is able to recognize that Kate is achieving further
success when she says she is able to come to the next session on her own.
Mum does not come to the two remaining sessions.

Notice how the homework is given, and the response: the therapist
assumes that there will be moments when Kate is at a 6 or 7, and Kate
assumes that it will be easy for her to notice them. Homework needs to make
sense to the client, and the best assignment here is the simple task of
observing improvements. The therapist can then ask what Kate notices she
is doing that is different at these times.

Key points

- Normalizing
- Compliments
- How has she found the session useful?
- What will she be doing differently?
- Observation task

Summary

Kate describes her problems and goals as she sees them (rather then how
her mother sees them!). The therapist asks questions to help Kate clarify her
goals and identify exceptions, and uses scales to help determine what the
next small step might be. This removes the focus away from Kate's biggest
fear – the phone. Hopefully the transcript gives some idea as to how SFBT
techniques work in context and how the approach determines the language
used by the therapist. It aims to demonstrate that there are a number of
questions the therapist could ask in response to what Kate says. Above all it
tries to show that significant change can occur within a single session.

Chapter 5
Sue: 'I forgot about Parkinson's disease'

It has been our experience at the Chelsea and Westminster Hospital that working with clients with Parkinson's disease (PD) and SFBT is extremely useful. This is likely to be the case with other chronic diseases where the medical situation is not going to improve long-term and we are dealing with high levels of a depression. Dealing effectively with depression can depend upon the clients' ability to adapt and their attitude as to how they are coping, and this case study is a good example of someone looking at the exceptions as building blocks for solutions.

Sue has been seen as an outpatient for three sessions. She is 58-years-old, became a Buddhist 21 years ago, and has had PD for a number of years. She is referred by the specialist registrar for help with 'dry mouth symptoms'. Speech can be difficult to follow because of reduced lips and tongue movement; communication is sometimes further restricted by extensive limb and head movement, as well as a quiet voice.

In response to the miracle question, Sue describes a morning of feeling happy, listening to music and sorting out her kitchen cupboards. She would like 'to get out and about more', visit people, and go swimming. She has just started to go to the gym, and the therapist aims to build on this, as well as getting clarification as to what difference it will make to Sue when the miracle day is happening.

Sue establishes in the first session that she is at a 5/6 in terms of how life is generally. She is aiming for a 10. Her confidence level is 6/7, in that she feels she will be able to improve on that first scale.

Sue also talks about 'panic attacks'. There are moments when she freezes and is unable, for example, to get on the bus or through a doorway:

> Sue: I know there's the freezing associated with the medication, and then there's the time I psychologically panic and freeze. It's so embarrassing holding everyone up.

Exceptions focus on when she doesn't get these panic attacks (breathing deeply and listening to music help), and the times when she is higher than 5/6. She is able to see that 'it's about attitude of mind', and describes the evening before the first session – pre-session change? – when she is at a 9.5.

> *Sue:*   Yesterday I visited a friend who is Brazilian. I danced with her two-year-old son. It was fun. I forgot about PD.

This chapter will focus on the second session as an example of EARS – elicit positive change, amplify, reinforce and start again. It begins with the therapist thanking Sue for the phone call she made an hour after the first session: Sue told the therapist that she had successfully negotiated the revolving doors of the hospital *and* managed to get a bus home.

The second session

Exceptions

Therapist:	Did you get to the hospital okay?
Sue:	I took the bus.
Therapist:	I loved your phone call. Thank you.
Sue:	I thought you'd like to know that. It's a challenge just to go through the door. It's incredible. If I take deep breaths I get through it.
Therapist:	You're right; it [the door] rotates fast. So, you managed to get through the doors and got on the bus today. Good. So have you been getting on buses more?
Sue:	A bit. I've been stopping and starting a bit. I have to say to myself, 'I've been able to walk before ... I will be able to walk again'. I get going again. It's really a question of talking to one's mind. Take control of one's mind.
Therapist:	As you were saying last time: you felt it was an attitude of mind. It's how you do that. So you find that saying something to yourself, that works.
Sue:	Sometimes it works better than others, but it's consciously doing that, and not to panic. I also feel very embarrassed about that. Trying to get into a cinema door ...
Therapist:	It's stressful, isn't it?
Sue:	Yes, it is.
Therapist:	Is there any particular thing that you say to yourself?
Sue:	I chant: (*chants*). I do that silently in my head, and at home out loud. It activates strong life force, which eases the situation. It's incredible really.
Therapist:	That must be something you've been doing for quite a while. It's not a new thing. I'm sure it's helped you through other stressful situations.
Sue:	I've been chanting for 21 years. It's all about life force that helps you feel in charge of your life.

Therapist:	So it's something that's helping you be in charge of your life now, and before in the past as well.
Sue:	It's a battle. There are two ways of looking: forwards and backwards. It's no good looking backwards.
Therapist:	But it's easy to say, isn't it? So what else has been working well since I last saw you?
Sue:	I went on the exercise bike. It's exhausting but I know it's good for you. It was five minutes but felt a lifetime.
Therapist:	And that was helpful?
Sue:	The physiotherapist said it was good to do. It's okay.
Therapist:	Well, it's one thing doing it with the physio, but taking yourself to the gym and doing it on your own is quite another thing, isn't it?
Sue:	That's right.
Therapist:	Do you have an instructor?
Sue:	Yes.
Therapist:	That's one of the things you said you were thinking of doing ...
Sue:	Another thing ... I had a wonderful time at the weekend at this course. We had an entertainer. I was on the drums.
Therapist:	Really!
Sue:	A Nigerian member, he had some drums and I tell you, it was so wonderful. I'm seriously thinking of taking it up. During that time I didn't feel bad at all. I was thinking about what I was doing and the excitement of the whole thing ... it really shows, you know, when your mind is occupied ... then ...
Therapist:	It's like the last time you told me about how you were dancing with your friend's child.
Sue:	Yes. Yes.
Therapist:	Marvellous. Where was that [the course]?
Sue:	The Institute of x.
Therapist:	So that was something new as well was it?
Sue:	Yes. Fantastic.
Therapist:	Have you played instruments before?
Sue:	No.
	(*pause for drink*)
Therapist:	So how were you able to just go and do that? Was it in front of other people?
Sue:	Oh yes: 80 of us!
Therapist:	Gosh!
Sue:	Each area in London ... ten areas ... each one did an entertainment.
Therapist:	So you planned it beforehand.
Sue:	Yes, it was great fun actually.
Therapist:	So were you surprised that you did that?
Sue:	Yes. It was wonderful, amazing. Such fun.
Therapist:	So you're obviously somebody who takes new and uncharted steps at different stages of your life. Is that something you've always done?
Sue:	I've always tried to expand as much as possible. Yes.
Therapist:	I think what's impressive is that you're holding on to that ... because that's so important, isn't it? You're still the same person, and that eagerness and interest in other things means you can go on doing that.
Sue:	Yes. One finds with this disorder it's really important not to go under.

Therapist:	Yes. It's about recognizing how you ... like your words 'expand your life' ... because maybe you have to look at different things, take on new things, maybe give some up, but that's not necessarily a bad thing. One's still developing. Goodness ... you've been busy! So what else? Anything else?
Sue:	No. I don't think so.
Therapist:	You've obviously still got the good feeling about the ...
Sue:	It's definitely a challenge to come back home, and it's at that point then not to go backwards but to look forwards.
Therapist:	Yes ... It doesn't surprise me though that you told me all that, because you seem someone who does go forward. It's a skill no doubt you've always had.

When looking at the video afterwards, the therapist becomes more aware of Sue's last comment about the difficulty of adjusting to the realities of life at home. The most useful question here could have been to ask how Sue manages to 'look forward' at home. Instead the therapist becomes interested in the other people in Sue's life; who she's communicating with, and what support mechanisms she has in place. You will notice, however, that Sue brings up this topic again - the difficulty between feeling the highs and the lows - as she is obviously aware that it hasn't been sufficiently acknowledged.

The skill in SFBT is not so much about asking the questions, but in asking the right ones at the right time. The practitioner should be led by the client: the most useful question is dictated by the last response from the client.

Key points

■   What's been working well since the last session?
■   Compliments
■   What else?

Other person perspective

Therapist:	If I told somebody ... somebody who knows you well ... Who would that be?
Sue:	Probably my great friend, Richard. We went to drama school together. We're just good friends.
Therapist:	Would Richard be surprised (maybe you've already told him), that you went and played the drums, which you've never done before?
Sue:	I told him, yes.
Therapist:	So was he surprised, or he thought 'Oh no, that's Sue, that doesn't surprise me'?
Sue:	I think he's always surprised by the things I do.
Therapist:	If I had Richard here, and I was to ask him, 'Richard, how would you describe Sue?' what would he say? What kind of person does he see you as?

Sue:	I don't know.
Therapist:	Just imagine for a minute that he was here.
Sue:	Goodness ... um ...
Therapist:	I mean, he obviously likes you because he's your friend. I'm wondering what particular things he ...
Sue:	We make each other laugh. Tremendously.
Therapist:	So you make him laugh.
Sue:	Yes, and he makes me laugh.
Therapist:	He'd describe you as someone who's quite funny.
Sue:	Yes. He's also seen me get upset about things in the past. He's seen both sides of me.
Therapist:	Sure. He's seen you down as well. I'm just thinking of all the reasons why he likes you ... You're funny. What else?
Sue:	I care about him.
Therapist:	How does he know that you care about him? What do you do that tells him you care about him?
Sue:	We keep in close contact.
Therapist:	So you ring him up regularly?
Sue:	Yes. Yes.
	(pause for drink)
Therapist:	So Richard would say you're funny, you're ...
Sue:	I'm terribly dramatic.
Therapist:	Dramatic! Oh really! He likes that, do you think?
Sue:	I think ... to a degree.

Eliciting information about Richard has been useful as part of the therapist's aim to reinforce Sue's strengths, and establish who her 'communication partners' are. The therapist decides at this stage to ask Sue a scaling question as to where she feels she is compared to the first session.

Key point

- Reinforce strengths (other person perspective)

Scales

Therapist:	So ... if I were to ask you, thinking about last time, where you might be on a scale from 0 to 10. About two weeks ago you said you were at 5, and you were thinking about being at number 6. Where would you say you are now? Roughly the same, or after the weekend you're on a ...
Sue:	It's been a bit of a battle of being at a high, or not so high. I'd say about the same.
Therapist:	You're absolutely right. That's normal, isn't it – that we can have real highs [and lows]? What would you say the weekend was? That moment when you were playing the drum?
Sue:	Probably a 9.5.

Therapist:	Brilliant! 9.5! ... How did you know how to do that: be at 9.5? What did it take?
Sue:	One's got to be aware that there is a high like that but that one can come crashing down. That's the key to it: to stay master of ones life rather than one's life master of one's self.
Therapist:	So you're aware that things go up and down, [but] you're still able to say to me you're at 5/6. You're able to step back and say that there is a middle ground. Okay, let's look at the middle ground stuff because that's a good point; we could look more at the 9.5, but it's the everyday stuff that gets us through too.
Sue:	Yes, absolutely.
Therapist:	Is there anything else that you could be doing differently that would help you feel things were a little bit more ...
Sue:	I'd like to be doing some work again.
Therapist:	Yes, that's something you've mentioned before. Is doing some work quite a big step would you say?
Sue:	Yes. During the day I can get really grotty.
Therapist:	So ... actually starting the work. What number would that be? Would that be quite a bit thing to aim for, whatever the work might be? I'm thinking about how you'd be taking steps to get to that point ...
Sue:	I'd like to think about that. I'd like to change track and do something completely different.
Therapist:	So what would be the first thing you need to do to get going on that?
Sue:	I don't want to do make-up any more.
Therapist:	I mean a starting point would be thinking of the skills you have as a make-up artist that can be transferred to ...
Sue:	I think I'm good with people. I need to be with people. One of my friend's teaching refugees. It's very interesting.
Therapist:	Is that something you feel you'd ...
Sue:	Yes. Something with people.
Therapist:	I think you're absolutely right. It's about using the skills you know you already have from past work experience. So being good with people ... anything else? I imagine as a make-up artist you'd be good with your hands, but that may be a bit more difficult for you now.
Sue:	My hands are fine.
Therapist:	Okay. What else? How would you describe the job as a make-up artist? Is it something anybody good with their hands could do?
Sue:	No. It requires a specific person. The personality of the person is equally important because you're dealing with people who are very highly stressed, a range of people. You need to be a very calm person.
Therapist:	So you're a calm person. And I imagine you need a lot of patience.
Sue:	Yes; not to get phased out by things.
Therapist:	So how would one begin now, looking for a job?
Sue:	I know a bit about how to work a computer
Therapist:	Ah! ... Presumably you want to be paid for this work, or you could ...
Sue:	I could start as a volunteer, but I need to be paid.
Therapist:	So it's how you start that up. Volunteering, or doing a course ... What do you think?

Sue:	I don't want to spend too long training for anything.
Therapist:	What would Richard suggest you do? Would he be helpful in how you take the next step? Anybody else?
Sue:	I can't think of anybody.
Therapist:	Any place that you know of?
Sue:	I might ring up the people in the immigrants' place.
Therapist:	That sounds like a good idea. See what they say ... So you've got your plans of where you want to be going.
	I think another thing I was impressed by [in the first session] was that you felt your confidence level as a 6/7, in that you feel things could continue to move forward
Sue:	It is an effort.
Therapist:	Nobody's saying it's not an effort! It's about doing it at your pace ... you managing your life and feeling you have control over your life, as much as any of us can. You were saying last time about changing your consultant; steps you were taking down that road so you felt, as you were saying, you've got more support. So do you feel you have enough support?
Sue:	Talking with the consultant will be good.
Therapist:	What will be helpful about talking with the consultant?
Sue:	It's working with a consultant, isn't it? You have to work at equal parts, patient and doctor: it's a two way thing. It's also about feeling they understand about the medication. One can't burden one's friends with that kind of thing.
Therapist:	It's about getting as much as you can out of them [the consultants], and seeing whether there's anybody else you feel would help with that as well. Does Richard understand?
Sue:	He's not a Buddhist. So he doesn't see life the way I do.
Therapist:	So the Buddhism helps?
Sue:	Oh yes. Absolutely. Through this problem I can change my life. One can resolve the suffering and enjoy one's life. I have a great desire to help people who are suffering in the kind of situation I find myself in, to show them that one can actually change it.
Therapist:	Other people with Parkinson's disease?
Sue:	Parkinson's disease, or any other disorder.
Therapist:	Yes. You've got such a strong belief to carry you through. So how are you going to be doing that? Are you already sharing that strength with others?
Sue:	We're already doing an awareness campaign in England. A friend of mine and I are going to schools, and we've got a video about Ghandi, Martin Luther King, and our leader ... We also do a brief talk to sixth formers.
Therapist:	Gosh! So you're able to stand up and talk ...
Sue:	With a microphone!
Therapist:	How many people?
Sue:	About twenty people.
Therapist:	Being sixth formers, they're not an easy audience.
Sue:	There's one class of 15-year-olds too.
Therapist:	Goodness! So how are you able to stand up in front of all of these people and talk about this?
Sue:	It's a very interesting subject. They'll be interested.

Therapist:	It's not everyone who's able to do it ... But I remember you saying you've given lectures before. It's obviously something you know so much about.
Sue:	Yes, it's quite a challenge.

Some time has been spent discussing Sue's idea of finding employment. Whether she is able to succeed in this will be dependant on how strong she is physically, and on her ability to control the 'on/off' patterns throughout the day which is so characteristic of PD.

It is important to remember to distinguish means from ends:

> One way to derive a richer description of the preferred future is to ask what difference certain outcomes will make to the client. This means treating what they describe as the means to something else rather than as an end point. (George et al., 2003)

This prompts the questions:

* When you aren't having so many panic attacks, how will that be good for you?
* So you'll be sorting out the kitchen cupboards/ going out to work. What difference will that make to you?

Apart from the obvious answer regarding work (that Sue would earn some money, which she has indicated is an area of concern), there is the perception that she will be getting 'out and about more'. This is something she mentioned as part of the miracle day. Even if at present she is only able to work on the kitchen cupboards, she has told the therapist that this is an important goal; achieving it will help alleviate the low mood and the perception that PD has caused her to feel 'stuck' in terms of managing her life.

Key points

- On a scale, where is Sue now?
- Where would she mark last weekend?
- How will she know things have moved one point up?
- Existing skills
- Compliments

What has the therapist got so far from using the SFBT interviewing techniques in this session? She has obtained a number of important details about Sue, and ones that she might not have elicited from a standard case history form. She has developed a picture of how Sue is communicating outside of the one-to-one therapy session, and as a result of this will be able to work with Sue and look at how to help maximize communication further.

Sue has already shown that, working with a friend and a microphone, she is able to communicate to a large group. Becoming solution focused, she could use these resources in other areas so as not to feel that PD will make her 'go under'.

The last part of the session will be to reinforce the advantages of working with goals and to give positive feedback. Sue and the therapist work together on a care aim (see Chapter 8).

Reinforcing successes and strengths

Therapist:	One last thing then. Although you were referred to me regarding a dry mouth, we've not spent that much time talking about that, apart from possible effects of medication. What's happened is that we've been looking at the wider context and how you're managing generally. My belief is that that affects communication. If one's got goals one's going to be able to function as well as one can and help maximize how one's communicating with other people. That's the 'communication umbrella' as I see it. We [the therapists] give ourselves a plan to see where we're going, and it would be more meaningful if we did it together. For example, what goals would you like to put down here? *(both look at care aim form)*
Sue:	I used to be really good at speaking, and now I swallow my words.
Therapist:	So ... overall goal would be 'Sue will be communicating more effectively.' How would you know?
Sue:	Other people's reactions. I'd be able to read a long passage and it'd be less stressful.
Therapist:	So it's about level of stress?
Sue:	Yes.
Therapist:	What's going to be the first sub goal?
Sue:	I think breathing is important.
Therapist:	How are you going to manage that?
Sue:	Diaphragmatic breathing. A few times a day. Breathing exercises three times a day.
Therapist:	What does that enable you to do?
Sue:	I'm calmer.
Therapist:	So it's helping with stress. I'm linking up the task with the result of the task. You'd be doing breathing exercises to help with stress. What else?
Sue:	The telephone. I tend to panic if I can't get to the phone in time. It's crazy because I've got an answering machine. It's an immediate evidence of stress.
Therapist:	What would show you that you were managing that better?
Sue:	Just relax and take time to get there.
Therapist:	Would you be doing anything differently with the phone? What would someone else notice you doing differently with the phone?
Sue:	I wouldn't talk so fast.

Therapist:	You'll talk slower. Anything that would help you talk slower?
Sue:	Breathing.
Therapist:	Anything else? I can think of other things. One in particular I've read about ...
Sue:	Give me a clue.
Therapist:	It was about putting a note by the phone. What might it say?
Sue:	Slow down!
Therapist:	Yes! Do you see how just something like that might be helpful? 'Sue to slow down on the telephone – note!' *(SLT writes)* Anything else? We're looking at overall how we can measure your level of stress, and communicating more effectively. Anything else that can help you feel you're moving forward? What kind of time frame would you like to give this?
Sue:	One week.
Therapist:	Is that long enough? In terms of real evidence you maybe need to give yourself a little time. You don't have to decide that now ... I'm mindful you've been sitting in one place for an hour. In terms of tying everything together ... there's a lot of things you're doing to move forward. It's stuff that comes from your Buddhism, your beliefs ... better than any therapy you can access here with me! So ... just the question I think I asked you before. How's it been useful you coming here today?
Sue:	What's amazing is before I wouldn't have dreamt of coming here or talking about it. I was so horrified. Every time I came across something in the newspaper I used to tear it up and throw it in the dustbin. So to come here is a real change. I couldn't bear hearing about it, and of course wherever you go you hear something about it.
Therapist:	About Parkinson's disease?
Sue:	Yes.
Therapist:	So it's about acknowledging it.
Sue:	Yes. To find out about it. Rather than be a victim ... the fear was so great.
Therapist:	Yes. Coming here is just one of the many ways of conquering that fear, as you say.
Sue:	And you're so helpful. Fantastic.
Therapist:	You're a good communicator, so that's already there! So anything that you'll be doing differently when you leave this room? Last time it was the bus, the doors ...
Sue:	Go through the doors again. It's quite a battle really, in all sorts of things. It's winning over the situation and not be pulled down by things.
Therapist:	Yes. It's holding on to that. It's looking forward, and noticing when you are doing it.
Sue:	Yes, absolutely.

Although Sue has taken some medication during the session, her limb and head movement have become quite pronounced. It would not have been productive for the therapist to extend the session for another five minutes so as to give a better summary of the points that had come up during the session. Furthermore, the therapist is struck by Sue's comments on how she has found the session useful; not that they have been discussing work, how to improve communication or support mechanisms, but that Sue has found it helpful to talk and 'find out' about Parkinson's disease. The therapist's immediate perception of what they have been doing is quite different from that of her client. However, watching the video later, she realizes their goal is the same: to alleviate 'the fear' of PD and, by reducing stress, maximize Sue's potential to see and communicate with others.

As part of bringing the session to a close, the SLT highlights the episode goal as 'Sue will be communicating more effectively.' Better use of the telephone and better management of stress, combined with some strategies (not putting her hand in front of her mouth when she talks, for example) could lead to a successful outcome; Sue will feel she is communicating more effectively, even if there has not been a significant improvement in speech. She has also identified that she is 'good with people' and needs to be with them. Trying to ensure that this need is met can also be included in the goals.

Key points

- Reinforce goal formation (care aim)
- How has she found the session useful?
- What will she be doing differently?

SFBT has given the therapist and client the ability to discuss concrete plans and at the same time address some attitudinal issues. It has not been a session where Sue has listed the things she can't do and the therapist has listened, in the hope that once the client has poured out all the bad feelings there is more room for problem solving (which strives to eliminate the problem or replace it with more desirable behaviours, attitudes or feelings).

How much time to give to 'venting' is a topic frequently discussed in SFBT. Clearly the practitioner needs to allow time to find out what and how the client is thinking and feeling about certain issues, particularly in the first session. But it has been the experience of several clients that the more they vent their frustration and anxiety, the more frustrated and anxious they become. In SFBT the venting of emotions is not the goal or focus of contact; its purpose is to establish a working relationship, so that the practitioner and client can work together as soon as possible to look at outward signs of success. As they work on what is there, rather than what isn't there, the solutions emerge that help reduce the feelings of helplessness and being trapped. As Sue puts it 'not to go backwards but to look forwards'.

On a lighter note, in the next session with Sue, the therapist is reminded of the importance of collaborative goal setting. Sue talks about the need to get her confidence back, and not being dependent on the medication. Her speech is less intelligible; she is complaining of feeling weak, and is quite tearful.

Therapist: What would help you feel a bit stronger right now?
Sue: A cup of sweet tea and some chocolate.

There is a noticeable difference in communication after a cup of tea and a chocolate biscuit: Sue's body posture improves, her voice is stronger and overall mood has changed. When asked how she could use this to help her if she feels weak again she replies:

Sue: I could make a thermos of tea for when the life force drains away.

Sometimes the simplest thing becomes a possible solution.

Summary

Sue finds scales useful. She is able to identify the times when she can achieve a high level of success in how she is managing overall. Acknowledging the fluctuation between the highs and the lows, Sue focuses on her strengths to help define goals for the future. SFBT respects clients' goals by accepting that it is helpful for Sue to think about looking for a job (even if the therapist feels this may be a number 10 and unachievable). What is important is that Sue identifies that she wants 'to be with people' and they can both explore the times when she is achieving this, and they can also look to see if there is anything else she could be doing differently.

Chapter 6
Focused on families

Abundant information is already available from clients who stammer on how they view themselves and their relationships with others. More recently there has been a growth in the number of assessments and programmes that focus on the psychosocial effects on the person who has difficulties as a result of stroke, chronic disease or head injury. Material has also been produced by speech and language therapists that does not require sophisticated linguistic ability from the client and the VASES (Visual analogue self-esteem scale) is an example of this (Brumfitt and Sheeran, 1999).

A resource pack has been produced called SPPARC ('Supporting Partners of People with Aphasia in Relationships and Conversation') which is targeted at carers (Lock, Wilkinson and Bryan, 2001). It is based on interviews and assessments that include questions on feelings and emotions resulting from changes in communication.

There is no doubt that it is important to identify what and why attitudinal changes occur as a result of brain damage, and it is useful to discuss issues such as self-esteem, quality of life and role change within the family, particularly in a group environment. Results from the problem solving approach used in the SPPARC programmes (support and conversation training) showed positive outcomes, even when the person with dysphasia was not actively involved in the programme.

Through its focus on solution building rather than problem solving, SFBT can also help reduce the sense of disability and emotional consequences of dysphasia, and there is the added advantage that useful and workable solutions emerge that are not necessarily related to the problems. This chapter looks at the description of clients and their families and how they would like to lead their lives differently in relation to each other. It offers some strategies and techniques that practitioners can use when working with clients and their significant others. For example, if clients live alone, it is useful to ask the question: 'Who knows you well?' As you will see from one of the case examples, it may be the dog that becomes part of the solution.

Solutions in the present

1. Family member as expert witness

Practitioners can ask carers to notice the times when things appear better, and encourage this process to begin from point of contact. Working with a carer is particularly useful if clients find it hard to identify exceptions.

Case example

A woman suffers a stroke but her daughter is unable to visit the hospital. Now she is with her mother at home, and having a telephone conversation with the therapist:

Therapist: Would you like to bring your mother in [to the hospital] for an appointment?

Daughter: What exactly is speech and language therapy?

Therapist: Well. We'd be looking at her speech. Have you noticed any improvement since she's been at home?

Daughter: Yes. But it fluctuates. Sometimes it's good, sometimes it isn't.

Therapist: What about understanding?

Daughter: I've noticed if you stand in front of her ... if she sees your face ... it works better.

Therapist: Well. Those things that you've described are exactly what we look for. I always say *you* are the expert rather than us, as you're with her all the time. We can run through all of this in a session. Keep noticing what works and we can build on that.

Case example

A young man has not found any specific strategies to help with his aggression, which has become a problem as a result of a TBI. His carer is able to remind him that he recently managed a difficult situation when he did not get angry. It appears he was able to do this because he was tired and said to himself, 'I'm chilled!' He wants to practise saying this, and assigns himself this project to work on in the future. SFBT has helped him feel he has some control over his life, and both he and his carer are encouraged to keep looking for those 'sparkling moments'.

Case example

Shirley has had a period of intense rehabilitation following a severe subarachnoid haemorrhage. She feels her progress has plateaued, and her loss of confidence and motivation has prompted her to be referred as 'she is not letting her husband out of her sight'. Her husband is able to help Shirley identify the times when she is already feeling confident and independent: washing her teeth is indeed a small miracle considering her disabilities, and is only one of many tasks Shirley is achieving. Her confidence is boosted, and Shirley feels, 'I can do it!'

Key points

*   When do things work well at home?
*   When are the 'sparkling moments'?
*   When are the times that x can do things independently?

---

2. More compliments

Clients vary: some may depend on their communicative ability for self-esteem while others are able to see any deficits as having little impact on their lives. Compliments give encouragement to both clients and those involved in their care.

Case example

A man has been referred by a nurse specializing in Parkinson's disease for help with his speech. He feels his communication is okay and that he is managing fine. Do you persuade the client that he has a problem, and give him advice and information anyway? Compliments help here: first, to the nurse for picking up on any speech intelligibility and passing on the referral and secondly, to the client for managing as well as he is. The client is encouraged to ask any questions, and to contact the speech and language therapist in the future should he have any concerns.

Case example

Patricia is able to say 'Yes', 'No', 'Gosh!', 'Oh dear!', '12345'. Very occasionally other words (mostly names) can be elicited with prompting. Her facial expression, gesture and use of intonation are extremely good. However, five years after her stroke and having accessed a large number of therapists, Patricia is still trying to find a therapist who will 'make her speak' (points to mouth). She does not want to work on drawing, writing, the computer, or a communication book.

SFBT helps the therapist feel she had something to offer the client. Working with Patricia and her carer, the following points emerge in two sessions before she is discharged:

* Patricia puts herself at a number 6 on a scale of how she is managing overall. How has she managed to be at 6? She grits her teeth/clenches her hands to indicate that she is a very determined person. The therapist lists communication strategies that she is doing, such as good eye contact, good gesture and intonation, under the 6.
* When are the times communication works well? Patricia indicates the carer, the therapist, her family and on holiday. What is it about a holiday that means communication works well? Patricia indicates that she is thinking less about her speech.
* When are the other times that Patricia is thinking less about her speech? When she is reading, shopping, eating and at the hairdresser.
* What is the carer doing to help with communication?

Carer:	I've been with Patricia for four years – I know exactly what she's trying to say. She loves the phone and manages it very well. She has a good memory. I told her my name wasn't 'Yes', so now she says it. I give her the first letter and she can complete the word. (*to Patricia*) Where did we go on holiday recently? Sp–
Patricia:	Spain.

The therapist compliments Patricia on being such a determined person and having a good memory. She compliments the carer on using prompts that appear to help with word-finding difficulties by saying, 'I can see that giving the first sound of a word to Patricia is really useful.' She encourages them both to continue to use their resources and such useful strategies to facilitate successful communication.

3. Partnership

SFBT promotes effective working between couples when they may struggle to adapt to a new situation brought on by disease or a traumatic event.

Case example

The question 'What do you find useful?' gives focus to a couple who are trying to maintain a routine despite obstacles presented by Parkinson's disease. The husband is trying to get his wife to get out of the house more, but she is nervous of falls:

Wife:	I tend to feel it's a big issue going out.
Therapist:	What would make it less of an issue?
Wife:	If I set a time everyday. 2.00 p.m. would be good.

Case example

Another couple are finding communication difficult as a result of Parkinson's disease:

Wife:	(*to therapist*) Sometimes I ask him to spell a word if I don't understand, but I'm sure he finds it very annoying.
Therapist:	(*looks at husband*)
Husband:	No. I don't mind.
Wife:	And I'm always trying to encourage him to do things, but I don't want to do it too much.
Therapist:	Do you mind your wife doing that?
Husband:	No.

Some couples can get stuck in unhelpful dialogues. A young woman has been describing how her husband says things to help her find a word: 'He tells me to 'spit it out' and that really doesn't help at all'. The practitioner asks what he could be doing differently. She demonstrates how he would make encouraging noises or remain silent. 'He would be coaxing.'

A similar question was helpful to a man with a stammer, who likes to practise reading out loud. However, he is irritated by his partner who keeps interrupting him and telling him to slow down. What could they be doing differently? He decides that receiving comments when he has finished reading is more helpful.

4. Existing resources

Couples can adapt to new situations using their existing strengths and resources. Indeed, there are SFBT practitioners who believe that

> couples don't need to go to skill-building classes; they don't need to be 'fixed' or 'cured'. By redirecting people's attention to their innate strengths and abilities, many problems can be resolved easily (Weiner-Davis 1992).

This can be a comforting thought to practitioners when, as frequently happens, only one member of a couple attends a session.

Case example

Client:	I feel I'm 80 per cent on the scale, but my wife finds it difficult to follow my speech. I've seen today I'm avoiding noisy places, I'm able to slow my speech down ... I even know when my speech works best [midday, when he's not tired]. I'd like her to come here. She might see that I'm doing all the right things.

Family members or friends can give a description of clients as to how they were before physical and/or cognitive changes occurred, and serve as a reminder to all that there can be core elements to a person that remain unchanged.

Case example

Caroline is 40 years old when she has her stroke. Initially she can only communicate through eye-blinks, and two years on she still has significant communication difficulties. However, she feels she is at a number 6 because of the progress she has achieved. She is brought to the hospital by a girlfriend, who sits in on the first part of the session.

Therapist:	(*to friend*) Does it surprise you that Caroline has got all the way up to a number 6?
Friend:	No. Caroline has always been amazing. She's determined, stubborn, a chatterbox ... remarkable!
Therapist:	(*to Caroline*) Who else sees these things? Would the nurse at home say you were remarkable?
Caroline:	Yes!

This conversation clearly reveals Caroline's strengths and resources, and opens the way to further discussion as to how she has achieved past successes. By the third session Caroline makes no mention of difficulties with speech. Her focus has shifted to issues concerning her young daughter – normal parenting concerns.

Clients can be asked to imagine a family member or friend in the room who can list their strengths. Alternatively they can imagine their guardian angel, sitting on their shoulder, who is dictating a list of their positive attributes: which personality traits or positive beliefs 'do you value most and want to continue to influence your approach to life?' (Dolan 2000)

A young woman, who has a severe stammer, uses this technique to identify a number of qualities in herself. She keeps the list in her pocket so that she can refer to it when she needs help with positive thoughts and feelings about herself and which she can use to move up her (numerous) scales. 'If I think back to six months ago – it's incredible. Everything just snowballed. Now I've got a life.'

5. Other person perspective

Clients and their families bring with them their view of the situation. In SFBT you ask questions that invite them to a different view that might help them take new actions and construct further solutions. Clients may find it difficult entering another person's frame of reference, but it can often make a real difference to a situation where other strategies have not worked, particularly in the case of adolescents when they feel the problem is other people.

> **Key point**
>
> ■   Suppose your family/friend/dog was here. What would they see you doing
>   differently when things are slightly better/the problem has gone?

Case example

Kathleen has lost her confidence. She lives alone at home with her dog, and
because she now has fits as a result of her stroke, her loneliness is compounded
by her fear of leaving the house. She has problems processing language.

| Therapist: | After the session, what will your dog see you doing differently? |
| Kathleen: | I'm happy and excited. We would go to Brighton and run on the beach. |

Kathleen has some unrealistic expectations, such as wanting to drive again,
but they are able to look at small and achievable solutions that the dog might
notice as different.

'She has negative self-image and low confidence regarding communicative
abilities, and avoids social situations.' This is the note that is sent when
Kathleen is re-referred two years later.

She works on scales and the miracle question:

| *Kathleen*: | I can't expect to go to the top. That's good enough [7] considering. I don't think I'll ever be able to drive again because of the fits. On my miracle day, I don't think I'd be any different. |

Kathleen does not need to feel a sense of failure that she has come back for
assistance. It is quite possible that the previous intervention did not work or
last. It is also possible that new issues have arisen. The analogy of the doctor
is a good one:

> If you come in with a broken arm, your doctor X-rays and sets it. If the next year,
> you came in with a broken leg, the doctor X-rays the leg, sets it and sends you on
> your way, without necessarily relating it to your previous injury, except, for
> example, to rule out bone degeneration or domestic violence as causes.
> (O'Hanlon and Beadle, 1996)

In Kathleen's case, because of the neurological damage, her level of insight is
initially poor. In her second episode of care, her perception has changed and
become more realistic. The practitioner's task is to help her construct goals
that are as concrete and measurable as possible.

Case example

After a crisis when she thought she may have cancer, a young woman is still
concerned about her voice. Her husband does not see it as an issue. She is
helped by the questions:

* 'What does your husband need to see for him to realize this is a concern for you?'
* 'What will he be doing differently when he realizes this?'
* 'What will you be doing differently then?'

Case example

A client has Parkinson's disease, and his wife has brought him to be seen by a speech and language therapist so that she can understand his speech better. However, the client says he is not worried about his speech. The therapist listens to them both, and asks the client:

* 'Is there one thing that you could be doing differently that your wife might find helpful?'
* 'What could she be doing differently?'

These questions were helpful to all concerned, not least the therapist who felt she would have had some difficulty dealing with this situation prior to her training in SFBT.

It is useful to ask clients to report for another even when they are both in the same room. This is the case with Barbara, who is keen to re-establish her independence after a stroke but feels her daughter is being over-protective. The practitioner suggests:

* If I were to ask your daughter what she wants you to be doing differently, what might she say?

Barbara immediately says that her daughter would ask her (a) to take her mobile when she went out and (b) to promise to take a taxi home if she got tired. The daughter is pleased to see that her mother is aware of her concerns. It is evident that some change is needed; Barbara comes alone for the next session, and is looking forward to returning home on her own as a measure of her independence. At the end of the session her daughter arrives unexpectedly to take her back, much to Barbara's annoyance!

Self-esteem

'Self-esteem is strongly related to, but not equivalent to, depression and anxiety' (VASES, Brumfitt and Sheeran, 1999). Self-esteem has not been medically defined, unlike depression and anxiety, yet it is frequently damaged in people with speech and language impairments. Your view of yourself and your relationship with other people can be affected in all situations that involve communication, yet profound difficulties mean that traditional tests to measure this may be unreliable, or even too difficult to administer. In order to target this client group and measure self-esteem, Brumfitt and Sheeran developed the VASES: visual analogue self-esteem scale.

Having elicited the information, how do you work to improve issues such as self-esteem? Two case examples are given here which aim to demonstrate how SFBT helped the practitioner, client and partner, using the VASES as a baseline measurement.

Case example

Jack is 50 years old, in full-time employment, and lives with his wife and two young children. He suffers a left frontal-parietal infarct that causes severe expressive dysphasia, as well as moderate difficulties understanding what is said to him. Initially he is only able to finger point in hospital, but soon some words begin to emerge, and he is able to make all his needs and wishes known.

The speech and language therapist uses SFBT in hospital to highlight the times communication is working better: who, what, when, where, and how questions are used that are helpful to the staff and family. Once he returns home, issues around employment and role-change begin to emerge. Six months after his stroke his wife says: 'He's there, but he isn't there.'

The VASES is first administered four months post onset (Figure 6.1), and again seven months later (Figure 6.2). Nearly a year after his stroke you will notice an increase in positive scores (the positive responses sometimes referring to a picture on the left and sometimes a picture on the right, so as to avoid a bias as to how people respond to the VASES). Jack feels more cheerful, intelligent, and optimistic, and at the same time he no longer feels mixed up, trapped, or frustrated. The therapist congratulates him on achieving these changes, and spends time asking him how he has managed to do this:

Therapist:	What are you doing differently?
Jack:	I don't worry all the time. Don't get so frustrated.
Therapist:	What do you feel instead?
Jack:	I'm at peace. I'm lucky ... family ... just feeling you're doing something ...

You will also notice that Jack is more aware that he is not being understood at times and that he feels he is less outgoing. An increase in insight means this is a more realistic view, and Jack needs considerable support from his family when he is told he is not able to return to his job. Jack's wife is only able to attend a couple of sessions with her husband, as her own job and

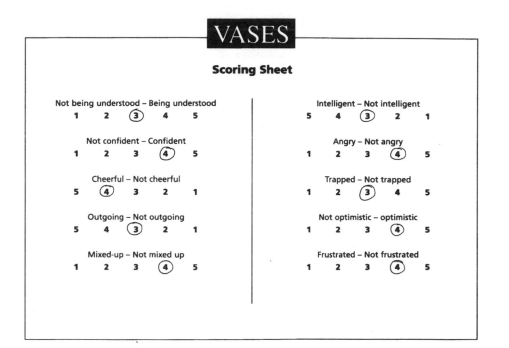

Figure 6.1 Jack – four months post onset

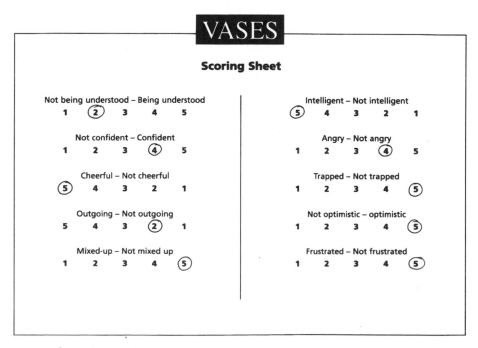

Figure 6.2 Jack – nearly one year post onset

home commitments mean there is little time left to come in to the hospital. She is adamant that she does not want to attend a group: 'I'm shy. I don't know if a help group would be okay for me.'

Lack of time and big issues to deal with – a familiar story for those in the health care profession, as well as for the clients and their families. Jack's wife is able to arrange a single session on her own with the therapist, ten months after the stroke occurs. The therapist compliments her on managing a difficult situation and they explore ways that could help her feel that the situation might improve further. Jack used to make the important decisions in the household; she feels that she is stronger than she used to be, and coping well with the role changes that have occurred since the stroke.

Key point

- Who, what, when, where, and how questions establish when communication is working well. These can be followed by compliments which help boost self-esteem in the client and family members.

SFBT recognizes the value of a single session, and operates on the assumption that therapy can be brief and effective. Jack and his wife are encouraged to contact the department again, but following the completion of the VASES for a second time no further input is requested.

Case example

> Wife: I know he has a degenerative disease but I wonder if there is a technique to learn to cope with the problem of not finding the words. He's lost his natural ability, but is there a recipe for coming to terms with it? I'm determined to help him live a decent life.

William's probable diagnosis is Lewy Body Disease; there is no 'recipe' for coming to terms with a deterioration in language which is likely to continue. However, SFBT can help him recognize that he is using all his skills and resources effectively to cope with the present situation, and enable his wife to feel that she is providing him a 'decent' life.

When William completes the VASES (Figure 6.3) his wife is surprised:

> Wife: I think you've only given a picture of communication with the speech and language therapist.
> William: No, I haven't. It's how I feel overall.
> Wife: (*long pause*) I'm aware I bring in my own frustrations here.

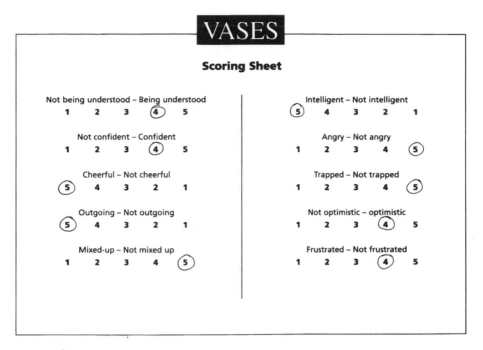

Figure 6.3 William

Although there are limitations in the overall research design, the study by Lee (1997) provides evidence for the assumption in SFBT that 'both problems and solutions are subject to a person's construction and interpretation, [and] the relationship between problems and solutions is not one to one. Goals, as such, need not be directly related to presenting problems.' The goal for William's wife becomes one where she will look at the times that she is slightly less preoccupied with the status quo and think about what further support mechanisms she might find helpful.

The situation is quite different five months later; William is admitted to hospital, and there is a marked deterioration in his language skills. He tells the therapist that 'It's all a bit of a swiz, and rather depressing.' The therapist uses coping questions:

* Things have been difficult. How have you been getting through?
* What do you do that helps you cope?
* What do you think your wife most admires about the way that you have been struggling with this?

A specialist nurse is offered to help support the wife at home but she does not feel she wants further assistance at that moment in time.

Solutions in the future

Miracles

A number of examples are given in this chapter that are concerned with exceptions; times when families are already making a difference. Hypothetical questions facilitate the development of a preferred future in as small a detail as possible, and help to ensure that there are shared goals. What you will notice is that regardless of the problem, the solution that clients describe is remarkably similar.

Case example

Joan feels her recovery has reached a plateau since her stroke two years ago. The physiotherapist feels she has unrealistic expectations regarding mobility and has suggested counselling, but Joan is not interested in this option. She agrees to a few sessions working with SFBT, however, and comes to the first session on her own. The therapist asks her the miracle question:

Joan:	I wake up and I can turn over. I can stand up and walk on my own ... I can get to the bathroom. I make breakfast.
Therapist:	What else?
Joan:	I'll be able to put my arms around my partner, Roy. He's wonderful ... he does everything.
Therapist:	How will you be feeling?
Joan:	Relief. I'll agree to go to the park and feed the ducks. I'll make steak and chips for him, and his favourite tomatoes with garlic.

The following week she comes back with Roy. They have been for a walk in the park, and her friends have noticed a difference in how she is coping generally. They are joking, touching and comforting each other throughout the session. The therapist asks Roy the miracle question:

Roy:	We'll get up. Joan can do her things, and then after breakfast we'll have a walk ... in the forest, by the sea ... There will be sun ... light.
Therapist:	It's interesting that you're both looking at the same thing; being together ... like a normal couple. How different is this from what you're doing already?
Joan:	I watch a lot of TV. I know Roy doesn't like me doing that but I don't want to bother him. I feel guilty watching TV though.
Therapist:	What would you like to feel instead?
Joan:	That I deserve it. So if I do some exercises first, then I feel I deserve a rest and I can watch TV.
Roy:	I saw my mother sit in front of the TV and die of cancer. I'm fearful that Joan will fill her brain with 'soaps' ...
Therapist:	(*turns to Joan*) How can you help Roy with his concerns?
Joan:	I'll do some ironing, read a book, wash up, try the computer ...

Therapist:	Gosh ...! And what can Roy do to help you with your concerns?
Joan:	He can show himself more self respect. Not always put everyone else's needs first.
Roy:	Yes. I know what I need to do. I need to lose weight. I've been bad-tempered these last two years. Angry.
Therapist:	What do you want to feel instead?
Roy:	Calm. I need to do things for myself. I need to get out ... have time out.
Therapist:	How confident are you, on a scale of 0–10, that you'll be able to do some of these things?

Joan does not feel she needs to come back for further input. Roy decides he would like to access further long-term assistance.

Key point

- What do you want to feel instead?

Case example

The theme of walks and dogs happens again in the miracle question with another couple. The reason for referral is to see if there is anything else they could be doing to help with some changes that have occurred in communication as a result of memory loss. The 59-year-old man has small vessel disease. After discussing communication issues, he describes his miracle day: 'I'll spring out of bed, maybe ravish her, go to the shop, take the dog for a walk ... sit in the sun.' What will she see him doing differently? 'He'll be up early, smiling ... he'll make me a cup of tea.' What will you do when he does that? And so on.

They are seen for a single session. They both know that there is no miracle that will 'cure' the memory loss, but through this questioning (How will that be helpful to you? What else? How will that make a difference?) they are able to establish well-formed goals that help maintain their hopes for the future.

If family members have perceptions that conflict with each other it is important to work towards a joint definition of goals and a joint solution:

> respectfully explore the perceptions of the family members who are stirred up, asking them what they think will be different when the problem is solved ... notice what clients are already doing that is useful to themselves, and helpful to their significant others and compliment them for those actions. (De Jong and Berg, 2002)

An example of this is a mother and son (aged 20) who come to therapy for help with his stammer. He wants to improve his speech but feels that at work he is 'normal': 'I'm up for a laugh, take things as they come.' His miracle day would be much the same as usual except that 'my mother wouldn't be nagging me'. His mother says 'He never says anything.'

The practitioner listens to the mother's concerns, notices what she is doing that is useful, and compliments her on being such a caring person to her son. By rephrasing 'nagging' as 'concerned', and 'wanting the best for her son', the two family members are able to see new and different ways of behaving.

Scales

Self-rating scales give an idea as to how the clients evaluate progress made, and how they will identify future signs of progress. A score of 10 (where 10 equals the miracle day or when the problem no longer has an impact on their lives) suggests a positive outlook and no need for further input. It might also suggest lack of insight when dealing with clients who have cognitive deficits.

Case example

Julie is keen for her friend to have ongoing help after her stroke. The client had indicated when leaving hospital that she did not want further assistance, but Julie is convinced that changes can be made if regular, intensive therapy is provided. She brings her friend in for outpatient appointments but progress is minimal; due to poor comprehension there is little carry-over from activities, even when they are focused on functional activities at home.

Julie rates her friend's communication skills as 6, while her friend marks 10 on the scale (where 0 shows a sad face and 10 shows a happy face). Through the use of scales, Julie is able to understand for herself that her friend's perception is quite different to her own. She is complimented on all the time and effort that she is providing, and is asked to contact the department again should she notice any change in the future.

Solutions are frequently unexpected. Another lady, 91 years old with a recent stammer where she is 'fighting to get the words out', feels she achieves a number 10 when she helps out at the Day Centre. She goes there twice a week: 'I don't stutter at all. They don't want anything from me. I feel so lucky when I look at the others. I feel useful.' Her son knows she likes to keep busy (she used to help his father with the family business), and has brought her a sewing kit. She's not interested in this: 'It's unfinished. I don't think I'll finish it. I don't feel like it.'

Six months later, the practitioner makes contact to see if any further input is needed. Her son rings:

Son: It was very useful coming to the last session with my mother. I was surprised when she mentioned the Day Centre. I suggested she helps out three times a week, which she does now and loves it! She feels she doesn't need to come and see you again.

Making home visits

Clients may be admitted to hospital, be referred as outpatients or, if they are unable to get to the hospital, be seen at home as domiciliary patients. There is often the perception that domiciliary work is particularly challenging; the clients can have complex needs, and it is difficult to discharge them when their needs are ongoing.

SFBT helps with maintaining boundaries. As Insoo Kim Berg and Karen Jick point out in their audio recording 'Making Home Visits' (Berg and Jick, 1995) 'we want to change people's lifestyles, and they haven't asked us to do that!'

Key point

■   The role of the professional is to assess risk and help clients identify meaningful goals, and these goals need to be what the client wants, rather than what someone else wants.

There does not need to be a special format for home visits that is different from that used with any other client group. You need to listen to the client's answer to the miracle question and see what bits of their miracle have already happened, look at scales and see how they are managing to cope, and ask how they will know that things are starting to improve.

SFBT helps the client focus on small steps and goals that they can achieve in a short space of time. The focus is on getting started in the right direction and noticing times when small miracles are already happening. It is based on the belief that a positive change in one relationship will have a ripple effect on others, and that the clients are part of the continuous process of change.

Scales can be used to facilitate the end of therapy:

*   Suppose 10 represents the end of therapy in three months' time/how you want your life to be. How close are you to that?

If they are still at number 7 in three months' time:

*   What do you need to keep doing to reach that number [10]?

Families and friends can be involved in reinforcing clients' resources and seeing ways that life could be different. They are given credit, and more importantly learn to give themselves credit, for finding useful solutions. 'In any field of work where deficit and loss of function are the focus of referral, an approach that can effectively transfer attention to achievement and growth is worth close consideration' (Iveson, 1994). This is always worth remembering when home visits require lengthy assessments that focus on deficits rather than clients' resources.

A therapist working in the domiciliary setting commented on SFBT:

> It helps me see that there are techniques that can turn our assessment process around a little and make the process less wieldy. For some of my clients, completing the whole assessment process first is unrealistic. I feel I have to do something in the first session to help support my clients in the difficult situation they are in.

A case example illustrates some of the points made above.

Case example: Hazel

78-year-old Hazel has returned home to live with her disabled husband following her stroke. Although she is independently mobile, the community team feel that 'her severe anxiety and frustration will impact negatively on her rehabilitation'. Hazel has had some counselling in the past, and she now agrees to some SFBT sessions to see if they can help with her anxieties.

Session 1: The therapist arrives to see Hazel at home, and is escorted up a steep flight of stairs to a cramped flat. There is a 'home help' in the living room vacuuming the carpet so Hazel and the therapist sit in the kitchen away from the noise:

Hazel:	I'm not in control of my house any longer.
Therapist:	Thank you for letting me come to see you. It's very comfortable here in the kitchen. (*Sees a large number of photographs stuck on the wall.*) Gosh! Are those of your family?
Hazel:	(*smiles*) Yes. I've got twelve grandchildren and two great-grandchildren!

They spend some time talking about her family. The therapist explains why she has come, and asks Hazel to complete the VASES. She appears happy to do this, but then gets agitated once she has completed the form:

Hazel: Come on, come on. I don't want to analyse myself. I want to get this finished. This is winding me up.

Therapist: *(looking at the VASES)* I'm sorry if you didn't find that helpful. It's helpful to me though because I can see that despite all the difficulties you've had recently, you're getting along pretty well. How have you managed to do that?

Hazel: I'm a coper. I just get on with it.

The session focuses on Hazel's strengths and resources, and looks at the times when she feels more relaxed and in control of her house.

Therapist: What one thing would make a difference right now?

Hazel: I haven't been out yet. I'd like to go shopping. I'd need someone to go with me.

Key points

- Explore solutions in the present
- Compliment
- Past successes help reinforce strengths
- Develop goals for the future

Session 2: The therapist rings Hazel's son and gives feedback on the first session. He says he will talk to his sister and the rest of the family. 'We can work on getting my mother to look at goals.'

Session 3: Three months on, and the therapist returns to see Hazel. The son is also with them.

Hazel: I feel on top of the world! Everyone understands me, and I've been getting out and about more. I'd still like to do some shopping.

Son: Mum, you already do some shopping.

Hazel: Yes, but it's only bread!

The therapist lists all the things that Hazel is doing to stay at a number 5 (on her scale). They include preparing breakfast and supper, tidying up after meals, washing up, hand washing clothes, and making the bed. They explore how she will notice when things improve further.

Session 4: Hazel has a telephone conversation with the therapist. It is three months since the second home visit. She says her speech feels 'much better', and that she does not need to be seen again. There is a slight improvement in intelligibility by the end of the conversation; Hazel responds to the praise and encouragement the therapist gives, and acknowledges that she has been able to monitor progress for herself. She is particularly pleased that this has been achieved after only a couple of home visits.

Key points

- Elicit
- Amplify
- Reinforce
- Start again

Summary

Chronic disease or neurological events cause change within the dynamics of a family and SFBT can help identify competence within family members to deal with change. Together with the client they can imagine the preferred future and use scales to establish goals and measure positive change. The therapist can compliment family members/carers/friends on their achievements and ask questions that invite them to construct further solutions. There is often the perception that clients who require home visits need long-term input; SFBT helps practitioners work in a collaborative way with the clients and/or their carers which challenges this viewpoint.

Chapter 7
Focused on groups

What would you like to have happen as a result of attending this group?
What are some of the goals, hopes and dreams for which you want support and
encouragement from the other group members?
Of these, which goal would you like to begin with? (Dolan, 2000, p. 143)

Solution building questions invite clients to re-examine how they see their
problems, and show that conversations themselves can lead to change.
Because SFBT assumes clients' competency in being able to determine ideas
and strategies for their lives, it moves away from a total dependency on
having a therapist 'do therapy'. Remembering this competency helps you
learn the power of silence when facilitating a solution focused group. Clients
are given the time to come up with their own strategies rather than the
therapist being the expert in devising a treatment plan.

This chapter will look at how SFBT has been integrated into two different
types of groups that are run at the Chelsea and Westminster Hospital. Linda
Metcalf and John Sharry have written in great detail on solution focused
group work, and examples of therapeutic groups and contexts will be
explored using the heading given in the latter (Sharry, 2001): these are single
session groups, planned short-term and topic focused groups, integrated
solution focused groups, organizational consultancy/team building and
teaching/training groups. There will be a discussion as to how the SFBT
approach works within a multidisciplinary team that follows a traditional/
medical model, as well as comments on frequently asked questions in
training to do with perceived problems in using this approach with clients
who have physical or cognitive difficulties.

Single session groups

The assumptions of a solution focused group are to help normalize
symptoms and create a sense of universality, as well as trusting that clients, as

experts on what works for them, can share this expertise with others (Vaughn, Hastings-Guerrero and Kassner, 1996). The inpatient group discussed by Kay Vaughn and colleagues has already been mentioned earlier in the book, but it is worth looking at some of the details to see if they have an application in other hospital environments with different client groups.

The groups at the Colorado Psychiatric Hospital have an open membership due to rapid client discharge, and include clients at various level of functioning with different diagnoses. Two nursing staff members lead each group, which lasts for one hour and takes place every day. Although every group is organized with a specific theme, the client's agenda may be generalized to allow all group members to benefit from the discussion. The type of questions asked might be focused on how they have managed in the past to overcome 'common stressors' and what coping strategies they have used.

The problem with clients who have suffered a neurological event is that this may be entirely new territory for them; they may never have been in hospital before, let alone had to deal with lack of movement in their arms and legs or difficulty using their speech apparatus to communicate. There may be the perception that it is beyond their control to change anything or that it is down to the amount of therapy they receive as to how much progress is made. The key is to enable them to see that their experience as human beings who have overcome obstacles in the past has given them strengths and resources to deal with current difficulties.

Questions that help create solutions

- How can I/we be helpful to you?
- How do you usually handle difficult situations?
- What difference will it make when you are able to talk/think a bit more clearly than you are now? What will you be doing?
- When is communication already working a bit better?
- Suppose tonight when you're asleep you're able to realize a big change in the way you're handling your situation. What would be the first thing you'd be doing differently when you wake up tomorrow?
- On a scale of 0–10 where 0 is the worst life could be and 10 is the best, what would 10 look like? Where are you now? How will you know you've moved up to ...?

You will notice that the practitioner is able to work with the notion that the disability may not go or even improve. What is important is the client can work with the areas they can control and effect change; it is failing to cope with the disability that so often causes depression rather than the circumstances themselves. This is seen every day in hospital where some clients are able to deal with severe disabilities while others with minor difficulties are unable to identify achievable goals.

Questions that help maintain progress

- How can you maintain the progress that you've made here outside of the hospital?
- How do you get through the difficult times?
- How will your partner/best friend notice that things are moving forward?
- Suppose you reach your goal. What will be different? Who else will notice?
- What particular qualities do you have that helped this to happen?
- Suppose it didn't happen. What would be the best you could hope for?
- What will you notice is different in 3/6/9 months?

These questions help clients maintain a conversation that is solution focused. Clients are not forced to 'accept' their disability (which can convey the feeling that they should give up on trying to improve their situation); the group works on realistic hopes which may help diminish the problem. The practitioner can highlight how one change in the client's life can have a positive impact on other areas seemingly unrelated to the problem.

Kay Vaughn and colleagues follow the framework given in Chapter 1 that suggests that the end of the session consists of compliments to group members on their coping skills and creative solutions. Clients are encouraged to compliment each other and to summarize what they found important during the group.

SFBT can be effective in the inpatient group setting as well as on an individual, couple and family basis. Successful implementation requires some training and supervision of staff; an example of this will be given later in the chapter.

Planned short-term and topic-focused groups

These groups last a defined number of sessions and have a homogenous client group. Initially, the example given here was not structured around solution focused exercises, such as the miracle question or exceptions, but it has evolved to adopt this framework. This change is described in some detail so as to help those who perceive major difficulties in taking on a SFBT approach in the hospital setting; the changes happened gradually because the speech and language therapist's (SLT) confidence developed gradually (in applying a solution focused approach to the group setting), and because the group needed to accommodate other presentational styles.

'Parkinson's Disease Education Group'

This group was established at the Chelsea and Westminster Hospital in 1998 by the physiotherapist, occupational therapist and SLT. The aim is to help provide their clients who have PD with further advice and information in a setting where they can meet other people with a similar diagnosis.

The group has a maximum of twelve participants (these can include partners/carers) and consists of a two-hour session each week, with a break for tea in the middle. There are two requirements for those who have PD; first, that they have a sufficient level of mobility to be able to come in to the hospital and second, that they have the cognitive ability to be able to benefit from attending the session. The group is set up in collaboration with the consultant involved in the PD caseload, and the six-week programme includes input from the three therapists mentioned as well as a dietitian, pharmacist and speaker from the Parkinson's Disease Society. To date eight programmes have been run.

'Managing Parkinson's Disease Successfully'

It is widely recognized by client led groups that they need to begin with a positive identity and a focus on the solution. Feedback from the participant questionnaire at the end of the first six-week programme is positive. It is evident that the general level of knowledge about PD is good:

* 'I thought it might be patronizing but it wasn't. About 80 per cent was reinforcing what I already know, and then there were some new things that I learnt. It was good listening to other people's experiences.'

Focusing on 'what's working' should apply to how the therapist approaches the therapy process as well as how clients and therapists solve problems together (Sharry, 2001). It is decided that the name of the group should be changed to 'Managing Parkinson's Disease Successfully'. The programme remains the same, but the title is a better acknowledgement that 'education' is only part of the reason why the clients come to the group.

Feedback at the end of the next programme picks up (unsolicited) on the name of the group:

* 'The title is very good. "Managing PD Successfully" is much better that the therapist oriented title of "Parkinson's Group" or "Parkinson's Education Group".'

Psychosocial issues

When starting a group, it is common practice to brainstorm expectations as to what the group members hope to get out of attending the sessions. Their goals are written on a flipchart, and it is referred to when the programme finishes to check that expectations have been met and to discuss what the next step might be towards meeting their goals. Even before the change in the name of the group, and despite a clear introduction as to the time limitations and planned programme with guest speakers, the hopes of the clients are far-reaching. Here are some of the expectations expressed by clients over the past seven years:

* 'Hope to feel differently about PD'
* 'To learn how to live with it (mentally/physically)'
* 'Hope for a better quality of life'
* 'What to expect in the future'
* 'To get motivation'
* 'To know how to cope'
* 'How to help the carer'
* 'To find out how other people cope with PD'
* 'To find out how it affects your mind ("it scrambles")'
* 'How to deal with the "there, there" factor from other people'
* 'To find out what's useful/not useful to say/do to others'

In 1998 it is felt that the group is not able to address these issues in any depth. By the time the problems and complaints have been heard (which dominate the discussion part of the programme), there is little time left to look at solutions, other than those 'taught' in the group. The problem talk is the central focus of the conversation rather than more of what is wanted to move forward; solution talk.

There is no doubt that the problem talk is helpful to some extent. It helps the clients feel that they are not the only ones with the problem and this provides a bond between them. It keeps expectations real as to what can or can't be changed. One woman (who takes 16 tablets a day) comments to another member (who takes 18 tablets a day):

* 'I've never met anyone who takes as many tablets as me. You've made my day!'

However, feelings of despair and helplessness in the face of a progressive disease can be exacerbated by too much problem talk, and this is the reason why some clients refuse to attend the group, saying it would 'only make me feel worse'.

> The balance between hearing clients' stories and exploring clients' goals is the art of leading a solution-focused group. Forcing clients to move too fast can actually prolong their need to convince you of the severity of their problem. Summarizing clients' stories and restating what you believe are the clients' goals help the client to feel understood. (Vaughn et al., 1996, p. 5)

With this in mind some of the programme is restructured. The SLT continues to give a presentation about communication and swallowing difficulties associated with PD (given on two separate days) and gives the same amount of handouts for reference, but the didactic part of the session becomes shorter. As a result of this shift in emphasis, the majority of group time is kept within solution talk. It has been suggested that 'a well-functioning solution-focused group spends 80 per cent of session time in solution talk and the remaining 20 per cent in problem talk' (Sharry, 2001).

Feedback from the group reflected this change:

* 'It was really excellent and just what is necessary to dispel some of the fear, ignorance and isolation which tends to be associated with PD.'
* 'Well organized – content pitched to include positive contributions from participants. Very upbeat. Good group management skills resulting in even contribution from members.'
* 'Suggest you keep the informal approach which is excellent.'
* 'More group meetings for our encouragement.'
* 'It was very useful and rewarding. The course exceeded my expectations.'
* 'It's the tips from other people, talking to other people who have PD.'

Key points

- The name of a group can be solution focused
- There is always the opportunity for solution talk

Solution talk

A change in group focus does not have to involve using SFBT techniques such as the miracle question. Simply the attitude of the practitioners, who see their role as identifying clients' strengths and resources, can influence a change in how clients relate to each other, and how they view their disease.

There are a number of ways to promote client competency:

1. Begin the programme by acknowledging that major difficulties exist. In the case of PD, symptoms may give rise to problems with mobility, balance,

aching muscles, tiredness, dribbling, speech difficulties, illegible writing, sweating, difficulty chewing and swallowing, constipation, memory problems, blank facial expression, uncontrollable tremors and depression (Swinburn and Morley, 1996). What is important is that not everyone develops all the symptoms, which are mainly tremor, slowness of movement and rigidity. The clients are the experts; they know which symptom predominates, when a new symptom develops or when the medication is not working. Congratulate them on recognizing the value of coming to a group, and on making the effort to negotiate transport and regulating their medication so as to be able to participate. Explain that time will be spent looking at the problems, but that the focus will also be on looking at solutions.

2. When talking about swallowing difficulties, the SLT would frequently be told by the group members that they do not have a problem with eating and drinking. Some members take longer to eat their meals, some avoid certain food because it is difficult to chew, but feedback suggests that a lengthy discussion on all the difficulties associated with PD and swallowing is not felt to be a priority.

The SLT asks herself what she could do differently, and changes the type of questions she asks. Previously, she had outlined possible problems to look out for, made available various handouts, and asked the group coping questions to elicit solutions. She now decides to ask the clients to go in to smaller groups to discuss the following:

*   What do you enjoy eating?
*   Discuss a really good meal you had recently.

It is explained that these discussion points are based on the assumption that the group members have always enjoyed their food and that they have found ways of continuing to do this successfully. The groups not only have an animated conversation about food and drink, but also give feedback on a number of solutions:

*   'I go to bed with a tray of goodies for nightime – chocolate, juice, fruit ... It helps with attitude.'
*   'Chinese food is good. You can pick some of it up in your hands and not worry about cutlery.'
*   'I eat when I want. I ignore the clock.'
*   'I go to a lovely restaurant where the chef cuts up the food for me.'

* 'When I eat out I scan the room for the best chair for me. If there isn't a good one I ask the restaurant to give me a kids' cushion to sit on. Then I can enjoy my meal.'
* 'I take my own cushion or leave one there.'
* 'I go out with my pills in a fly-fishing box as it just has a lid and then compartments inside. The docket box is fiddly.'
* 'I have a knife in my handbag for restaurants – it helps me cut things more easily.'

The last group member may have problems if she forgets to take her knife out before trying to board a plane! The point of listing these comments is that any therapist/dietician will recognize that they include many recommendations made as to how to make eating and drinking more successful; correct positioning, easier consistencies, useful equipment and frequent meals. The clients are the experts.

3. Solution focused questions can also elicit useful information when addressing communication. Common complaints with PD is that the voice quality is changed and /or quieter, and speech is slurred.

Therapist:	When is your voice stronger?
Client:	First thing in the morning.
Therapist:	What about saying the words? When is that easier?
Client:	When I'm relaxed.
Therapist:	What are you doing then – when you're relaxed?
Client:	I suppose I'm speaking more slowly.
Therapist:	What else helps with speech? What about saliva?
Client:	If my mouth isn't full of saliva it's better.
Therapist:	So what could help with that?
Client:	If I swallow first and clear my mouth.
Therapist:	What else? When are the other times communication works well?
Client:	When I feel well in myself. When I'm not lying down.
Therapist:	So when you're sitting upright it's better ...

In a group setting the practitioner can use these questions as prompts to get the members to discuss solutions they have found that help with communication (EARS). Again, the information has been gathered in a collaborative way, and can be reinforced with a handout later in the session.

> **Key points**
>
> - The clients are the experts on managing their symptoms
> - Compliment clients on the times when things are working well
> - SFBT promotes collaborative work

Solution techniques

As a result of these changes the SLT is feeling more confident in her approach, and has positive feedback that the group members feel that they are learning more about PD and that they are also feel that more of the attitudinal issues are being addressed. In the next programme she incorporates more SFBT activities.

> **Eliciting strengths in the group**
>
> - What's happened between when you woke up this morning and now, that tells you it's good to be alive?
> - Tell the person next to you about a project that you're working on, or have worked on in the past, that you're pleased with. What skills do you possess that have enabled you to make it a success?
> - Between now and the next session look out for something that works well in the week.

Responses to the last exercise are as follows:

Client A: I went out to an evening at the Arts Club. I was amazed. I don't go out much now [since I was diagnosed with PD], but I loved it. I listened to jazz and I even jived with someone. It was great.

Client B: I went to x [name of department store]. I noticed a pourer. I thought it would work really well for me to use with milk powder, and it saves me screwing the lid on and off.

Client C: I decided to do something about this flooding drain. I went to the council and got a very nice man. Now all the neighbours are organizing a meeting to discuss the issue.

Client D: I found out (actually I already knew, but hadn't got round to using them) that there is a taxi service called x. You dial from your mobile phone, and they'll come within minutes.

Client E: I have brown fingers. But a tree on my patio had a flower. I was really pleased.

Client F: I decided that if people say to me: 'How are you?' I will reply: 'Much blessed'. It avoids those long conversations where people have to talk to you about your health, or you say: 'Fine'.

The SLT makes some comments on these responses. She says that she is not surprised that they have done all these things during the week; a focus on what is working well enables people to find solutions for themselves without therapy input. *They* are the ones who are doing all the work, and as one member said: 'Something learned is not normally affected by PD.' Client A already knows how to jive, and that knowledge does not disappear just because he has PD. Client B and C are resourceful people.

Client E is a carer, committed to the full-time care of her husband who does not attend the group. The SLT suggests that this is the first time that she has talked about herself to the whole group, rather than being focused on the needs of her husband.

Scales

- On a scale of 0–10 with 0 being you feel your communication isn't working well at all/it's the worst things have been and 10 is when you feel it's pretty good/things are at their best, where would you say you are now?

The SLT introduces this: she tells the clients that she thinks they are all really good communicators from the evidence she has in the group, but in the end her rating is not what is important. What matters is how *they* feel about their communication, and a scale will help them decide where they are and what they can do to move forward. You may be surprised at clients' responses as to where they mark themselves on the scale, as well as the goals they give for the future:

* 'I feel like I'm already at number 10. I have friends, I go out ...'
* 'Since my diagnosis [of PD] last year my memory seems to have got better. Perhaps it's the medication.'
* 'I'm trying to be more selfish. Get a more minimalist life, scale down. I'm moving ...'
* 'I want to write this novel – I've got two already in the bottom drawer!'
* 'I want to do more things that are interesting. I miss that since I retired. I want to learn German, go to Germany and live there. Teach English in return for my lodgings.'

When the therapist asks the last person whether going to Germany is maybe a big goal, she replies:

* 'Yes, it is. What else would be interesting? I find reading difficult now. My memory is going ... I need to sort out my domestic life.'

She has now got some more realistic goals. Learning German and living in Germany can continue to be her dreams, and the therapist is not going to suggest they are unreasonable. In most cases, if you wait, clients will come up with achievable goals. If they don't you can say 'Okay, that's 10', find out where they are from 0 to 10, and work out what would be the next step on from where they are. This client is an extremely motivated lady, and another useful activity would be to scale her level of motivation towards achieving her goals.

The future

The group 'Managing Parkinson's Disease Successfully' has evolved from its original format seven years ago to one where the SFBT approach has been successfully integrated into the programme. The aim continues to be that of advice and information on PD from a multidisciplinary approach, but it has also become a group where the members are more involved from the beginning in formulating their own individual goals. Furthermore, between sessions they are able to work on techniques such as scales.

A questionnaire, which uses rating scales, is completed at the end of the six weeks. It provides feedback and helps ensure that the next group will continue to reflect the opinions of the group members as much as possible. One 'slot' that has consistently scored the highest score since the group began is the tea break; a reminder that it is not what the therapists are doing right but the effect of the 'positive, supportive interpersonal communication among the group members' (Sharry, 2001). This is a more likely explanation than a high rating of hospital tea!

Integrated solution focused groups

These groups are usually brief, and combine other therapeutic models; in the context of speech and language therapy this might include impairment work to focus on reading or writing, for example, where the clients have identified a need. SFBT can give some relief from problem talk and also provide a framework, as mentioned previously, for developing individual client goals.

The Chelsea and Westminster Hospital runs a group for outpatients who have dysphasia, held on a weekly basis, which provides a supportive environment to work on functional communication. It is run by an SLT and her two students, and has additional help from a volunteer. The group is small – a maximum of five members – and is aimed at clients who have some difficulties understanding and expressing language as a result of a stroke, but they are able to make their needs and wishes known.

Two SFBT group activities are described here, as examples of what might work with this client group. The current group members are Ana, Richard, James and Alan, and the activities are followed by more traditional SLT tasks for the rest of the session.

Games

■   A game can be helpful for groups that are difficult to get talking. One idea is given by Insoo Kim Berg and Norman Reuss in *Solutions Step by Step: A Substance Abuse Treatment Manual*. A pair of dice are thrown and the client answers a question that corresponds to the total of the roll of the dice. Follow-up questions clarify the answer and personalize the goal.

---

1.   Two sessions are begun with a question taken from the SFBT game:

Session 1

> *Therapist*:   What kind of help do people need from you so that they can communicate better with you?

Initially, Ana does not understand the question. She says she needs help with doing the shopping; when prompted, she describes how she will look at her 'food' picture book to get the names of items, so that she will have a complete list ready for the girl who does the shopping.

Richard and James have difficulty understanding people, especially if they speak too fast. Richard gets round this by showing people his stroke card, which asks them to slow down. He is prompted to use this successful activity with the telephone, which is an ongoing problem. He decides to keep his card by the phone so that he can read it out in times of difficulty.

James also has problems with the phone, particularly taking down names and numbers. He decides to have an alphabet/number chart by the phone so that he can follow the letters/numbers as people are speaking, and then copy them onto a separate piece of paper.

Alan did not attend the group that day.

Session 2

> *Therapist*:   When were you tempted to handle something the same old way and you said, 'No, I'm going to handle this differently'? What did you do?

Richard says that he is unable to give an example as he feels that if something works, why change it?

Ana says she might normally give up on something, but she now waits until she can ask someone to do it for her. Alan agrees. He gives the example of being unable to do his tie. Now he goes upstairs and asks a family member to help him.

Since his stroke, James has been practising reading out loud at home; he believes it has helped him improve his ability to say words. He used to ask someone to correct him if they were around, or he may have ignored his mistakes. Now he has a Dictaphone, which records his speech when reading. He listens to it while reading the target items, and attempts to self-correct when he knows the pronunciation is incorrect.

Key point

■　The therapist can compliment the group members on their ideas, and continue to encourage them to think in terms of other ways they can apply their skills. The questions promote an increase in client discussion and demonstrate the individual nature of solutions, while at the same time emphasizing the value of small steps.

---

2. The miracle question is used in the group; the therapist asks Richard the question and everyone listens to his response, which is then followed up with scaling questions. The aim is to get the other group members to think about their miracle question also, although they will not be asked in detail in the same session due to time constraints and the need for them to be given time to work on this.

Therapist:	... So how will you know this miracle has happened?
Richard:	Good heavens, how remarkable.
Alan:	That's a good day. That's what we all need.
Richard:	When I get out of a bed, I wouldn't have any problems with eat – wal – walking. Much the same. I wouldn't be speaking to anyone at that stage. When the lady comes to the flat, I've had dinner, no lunch – brunch.
Therapist:	Brunch or breakfast?
Richard:	Breakfast. I've had breakfast, that was all perfectly normal. I'd be speaking away without having to think about what one was looking at. I do some days anyway but if it's a really exciting question I wouldn't manage. That would be enough itself.

Ana:	That would be lovely, wouldn't it? It is a dream. I'm another person.
Therapist:	So what else will you be doing on this special day?
Richard:	I'm so old one doesn't need to do anything. I would go back to books. If I could eat - read, much earlier - easier. Walk a much larger dis - dis - distance.
Therapist:	What could you be doing now, from that special day?
Richard:	The main thing would be to read books. It's just newspapers, that's all I do, reading, writing.
Therapist:	(*drawing and explaining a scale*) ... Where are you now?
Richard:	(*points*) I should think about there.
Therapist:	What number would you give that?
Richard:	Oh, I should think a 4. I wouldn't know if a 5 or 4 ... a feeling. Writing would make a big difference - up to 9 or 10. I'm operating on all bits of me all the time. It's getting slowly better. Little bits of writing - odd words are better, but occasionally. Walking could be better, but it is better than it was. I do most things myself. My wife and I we used to operate together. But I can look after myself too. Shopping - I can do all that.
Therapist:	It sounds like you're a very independent person. Have you always been like that?
Richard:	Yes.
Therapist:	(*turning to the others and asking them to draw a scale*)
James:	I'm about here, at 85 per cent. You see sculpture was a goal. I could paint but I wanted to start sculpting. Also computing, walking. I go for walks, normally at least two times a day, twice a week, which is very important.
Therapist:	How have you managed to do all those things?
James:	I try for everything.
Therapist:	I know you find a tape recorder useful. What else do you find useful?
James:	I talk to myself. I have a book that I take notes in, not every day, but over the last three years. So I want to write a book about having a stroke. Write of my experience for all the other people ... I feel I want to help other people.
Therapist:	That sounds like a really good idea. What about you, Ana?
Ana:	I just keep getting worse.
Therapist:	Where would you be on your scale?
Ana:	Well I suppose ... (*places herself at 5*) I can still go and have a bath, a few things in the house, look after the cat. I'm not good at getting food. My daughter wants me to stay at home all the time. I haven't got anything to eat today.
Alan:	So what are you going to eat?
Ana:	I don't go out to get food. I want to go today. I'll get ... I can't remember the word - it won't come ... it won't come.

Some time is spent trying to elicit the word. Ana eventually remembers 'soup' at the end of the session.

Therapist:	What about you, Alan? Is there anything you can do to move up your scale?
Alan:	Tell me again ... no, I don't understand.
Therapist:	Take last week for example. What worked well last week ... something that you're really pleased you've been able to do?
Alan:	I couldn't put my socks on, now I can.
Therapist:	Wow! How did you manage to do that?
Alan:	All of a sudden I thought I can do that. I got fed up with everyone saying 'I'll do that' (*marks 'sock' moment on the scale*).

There is further discussion about what Alan finds useful in his life; this is a magnifying glass for reading, as he has poor eyesight due to diabetes. He begins to understand the way to measure change on his scale. The miracle question, the scales, and clarification of 'sparkling moments' take about forty minutes. The SLT could have asked Richard more questions on his miracle day when he said: 'I do some days anyway', or given Ana more compliments on achieving 5, despite her feeling that things keep getting worse. However, it is time to break for tea and continue with a different activity related to reading.

The group members find it difficult to mark change on their scales, but it is something to work on in the future, as well as asking the other members about their 'special day'. You will notice from the group conversation that there is sometimes the need for the solution focused questions to be repeated or rephrased. Repetition to help understanding is common practice for those involved with this client group.

Comments from the SLT students observing the clients are that Ana is unusually talkative and in a brighter mood than usual, and that they all appear encouraged by the positive feedback with regard to their achievements. It is suggested that the group members could begin each week by writing where they are on their respective scales using their own definition of success, and that the students could pull a theme from the comments made to discuss in the group. This would accommodate the occasions when clients are unable to mark progress, and coping questions could be used.

Richard dreams of being able to read books again, but what is interesting is that he is beginning to be aware that this is a very big step.

Key point

- By working on a continuum clients are able to take credit for what they have achieved and identify small steps, and they are not lost in a dialogue about absolutes (such as reading/not reading).

A solution focused approach is quite different to the medical model that 'plans strategies to solve the patient's problem by placing the patient in a structured group therapy' (Metcalf, 1998). There are benefits for both the practitioner and the client. As one therapist said: 'Since learning about SFBT I feel I don't have to 'cure' people any more. I know it's about what they do with their circumstances that really matters.'

Organizational consultancy/team building

Anyone who works as part of a team will appreciate how the solution focused model can be used to promote team building skills. Ben Furman, who works on 'ReTeaming', writes:

> Companies that have had the experience of working with well-known and expensive consultants say that solution focused therapy is better in terms of being more successful in furthering the development of good relationships among staff members. To perform such a feat, therapists can simply improvise and use exactly the same questions they use with clients. (Metcalf, 1998, p. 226)

SFBT assumes that the clients have the resources to help themselves, and that the practitioner helps them uncover, nurture, and use those resources as effectively as possible. In the world of business, traditional models have tended to assume that problems arise because there is some deficiency in the staff. As Louis Cauffman puts it, instead of giving advice and making suggestions, it can be more productive to ask solution building questions and elicit resources:

> Resources can be things as intangible as effort, motivation, loyalty to the company, collegiality, or expertise, but they also can be more concrete tools, such as communication skills, crisis and conflict management, procedures, business insights, technical tools, time, money, or attention. (McKergow, 2003)

Often discussions break down in the work environment because they revolve around too many labels and abstract concepts: $5,000 words or expert's jargon. It is the everyday language that can be more effective when working on specific goals or the '$5 words [which] are usually positive, detailed, and describe observable events and objects'. (Jackson and McKergow, 2002).

It may be that some terminology needs to be adapted to an organization's culture as senior executives could have a problem with therapy vocabulary as well as terms such as 'miracle'. An example might be 'A Letter from the Future' (Dolan, 2000). This is a useful exercise for clients who can imagine a point in the future; the problems have been resolved (or they have found satisfying ways to cope with them), and they describe how they have managed to do this to a close friend. The letter is not meant to be sent but to be kept as a record for themselves.

In a work environment, the scenario could be a meeting in four months' time when things have made a considerable improvement. What's better, who notices, what did everyone do to make it happen?

On a more regular basis, the agenda for weekly staff meetings can include a slot for 'activities of the week' in recognition that there are constant contributions from staff members to the department, however small. The use of scales can help with on-going issues and help clarify what would re-motivate the team or promote further learning. Performance appraisals can become a more collaborative process when looking at rating instruments: an example would be when employees are invited to rate their level of confidence in terms of their ability to improve on performance, or when they are asked to define their objectives more clearly and precisely (McKergow, 2003).

> What is a small step that you could make in the direction of the goal?
> What will be the first thing I (or another person) will notice about your therapy when it improves? (Miller et al., 1996)

Key point

- Asking yourself solutions focused questions and applying the principles to your own personal circumstances is an integral part of understanding and learning about SFBT.

Teaching/training groups

Comments are frequently heard that those who work in a solution focused way appear to remain more optimistic and energized than those who work from a more pathological stance. Even if practitioners work in an environment where a variety of techniques and approaches are used, they can insert language about strengths and resources into their conversation that make other professionals curious about the approach. It is a process that can take time and requires sensitivity, and SFBT needs to be presented as being one way of working among many.

An example of where this approach works might be an SLT working in a hospital ward. She is interested in finding out the times when communication is working successfully, and asks the staff to notice what the client is doing differently on these occasions. A process begins where staff start to notice other positive behaviours in the client, which is then extended to noticing similar behaviour in other clients.

However, increasingly SFBT is being taught in groups, and is used as part of the training in these groups. A study carried out by Bowles, Mackintosh and Torn (2001) on 'Nurses' communication skills: an evaluation of the impact of solution-focused communication training' is an example of this. The nurses and health visitors come from a variety of clinical settings, both in-patient and community based, that include surgical, medical, palliative care and family support. The training consists of four days over a period of eight weeks, and change is measured six months post completion.

Six areas are examined, four of which are competence, confidence and willingness to talk with people who are troubled, as well as the frequency with which the nurse speaks with people who are troubled. Baseline measures are taken using a Likert scale instrument; 0 equates to 'not at all [e.g. confident]' and 10 to 'extremely [e.g. confident]', while the intermediate scores do not carry a label (modelling the process of SFBT within the evaluation). There are methodological drawbacks in this study, not least the fact that the number of students is very small, but it is worth looking at some of the comments made.

Prior to the SFBT training, problem talk between nurse and patient places an emotional strain on the nurses:

* 'I dreaded clinic, because it was so depressing ... it was very much doom and gloom and problems.'

Even if her client has a chronic problem which she feels she is unable to change, SFBT now helps her

* '... balance it out with a positive, you know, "What's your good day like?" It makes, yes, it's lightened my load.'

Another nurse shows how she adapts SFBT to her client group:

* '... the miracle was how can we make this better? How can this be okay, this next period? What will make this feel more comfortable, more pleasant?'

Quantitative data show a significant difference in willingness to talk with people who are troubled; only one or two solution focused questions enable the nurses to engage with the clients more readily. There is also a positive directional change in competency and confidence, but interestingly a negative directional change in the frequency with which nurses speak with people who are troubled. Does this reflect a change in the perception of 'troubled', or are there fewer displays of 'troubled' behaviour as a result of SFBT? It may be the nurses are re-evaluating 'the extent to which they actually engaged with clients ... further examination of the efficacy of solution-focused communication in nursing is clearly indicated' (Bowles et al., 2001).

Key points

■   Change occurs through positive appraisal in the workplace
■   Formal training helps promote competency and confidence

What next?

*   'Do you have to be trained in SFBT in order to be able to do it?'

This was a question asked by a student who had observed a solution focused session with a client who had communication difficulties as a result of a stroke. She felt that the approach appeared simple enough but that it did not look easy to do.

*   'I get the feeling that I'll ask the questions ... and then what? How can I carry it through? Isn't this going beyond our clinical boundaries anyway?'

SFBT is about learning to look for client resources rather than learning about techniques. It is about learning to listen to the client, following the clients' goals and being client led. There may be 'typical' techniques, but all clients are different according to their own individual solutions and how they interpret the questions. Once students have learnt this, then the process has begun where they will learn and become more confident with each session.

The advantage of training courses is that the experiential nature of SFBT can be explored, and participants can engage in role plays and small groups where work and life achievements are discussed. Reading books on the subject or talking to others who work in a similar way within the workplace or on-line is enormously helpful, especially if there is little formal supervision or follow-up after a training course.

SFBT encourages the client and the therapist to feel resourceful. Some of the difficulties within a multidisciplinary setting are that professionals can get stuck within their areas of expertise, or that the clients' needs are left to be dealt with by another; the management of risk and need is something that care aims attempt to address (see Chapter 8) so as to promote collaborative teams.

It has long been the goal of training to get students to look at the 'whole person' so as to meet their clients' functional needs.

Client: This is not what I expected of speech and language therapy! It's
                 more holistic.

This is a client's comment on his therapy after two SFBT sessions. He reaches
a number 8 on his scale.

*   'How can you ask the miracle question if change is impossible because of
  physical impairments – with someone who has just had a stroke for
  example?'
*   'Aren't we forcing clients to say they've moved up a scale to show that
  therapy has been effective? What if the client can't find anything better?'
*   'I give practical strategies for when communication doesn't work. How
  does SFBT fit in with this?'

A SFBT conversation looks at clients' hopes and how these might be
achieved. It is understandable that after a stroke clients want their speech
and language back, or the ability to move their arms and legs normally. You
can say this is a reasonable wish. After accepting that, scales help clients
decide whether some hopes are more achievable than others, and they can
facilitate the process whereby clients come to the realization that there are
some hopes that are not realistic. In the meantime, they record the steps
already taken that indicate change.

Exceptions can usually be found if you look hard enough. If 0 represents
admission to hospital, there is usually improvement from that point in time,
however small, which can be linked to the client making an effort to
communicate, move or effect change over their surroundings. Coping
questions can help when there is the perception that things are not moving
forward (see Chapter 2). After having tried out some solution focused
questions on clients with cognitive difficulties, this is the comment from
someone on her second day of training: 'I asked about exceptions. All my
expectations were rubbish – they *were* able to focus on things. They made
goals. There was nothing for me to do! In the past I would have done another
Makaton [signing] course, but this time I felt they were managing perfectly
well with about five signs.'

Frequently the SLT tries to effect change by working on practical
strategies based on the times when the client's communication is not
working effectively. SFBT also works on practical strategies, but uses the
times when communication *is* working effectively to elicit these strategies.
Take the environment, for example. Communication can be difficult in noisy
surroundings, therefore the SLT recommends speaking in quieter settings.

Using an SFBT approach you would ask when communication appears to work well. This is a typical response: 'In the evening at home with my husband/wife. It's quiet ... no distractions.' It may become the goal of the client to ensure that these moments are extended, or that they keep that time for important issues to be discussed. SFBT 'fits in' comfortably with the therapists' case management.

* 'What about the medical criteria for success – what if this is different from the clients' idea of what they see as success?'
* 'What about progressive diseases? Isn't that a problem when you're looking into the future?'

Hopefully some answers to these questions have already been given in the book. They are questions asked after one day of SFBT training; there tend to be more questions than answers after this amount of time and subsequent days allow for case examples, further practice and consolidation. After a while the group begin to see that it is not so much that the medical team and the client have different criteria for success. Both want the client to achieve/maintain maximum independence and good health, but it is how they decide to get there that may be quite different. 'Both medical and social responses are appropriate to the problems associated with disability; we cannot wholly reject either kind of intervention' (WHO, 2002).

It is ultimately the clients' solutions that matter, so long as they are realistic and pose minimal risk to themselves or others. It may feel that you have to 'unlearn' some of the more directive approaches adopted by the medical model and it can require some courage to adopt the SFBT approach when this prompts questions from colleagues as to effectiveness. Talking about your own case examples and quoting research related to SFBT can be helpful, but the aim is not to antagonize the medical and nursing professions. It is about developing the skills and confidence of the workforce to deal with a range of issues without necessarily calling on the assistance of counsellors.

Training in the SFBT approach builds on your own personal competence and develops your skills in asking the most appropriate question. The more you use the solution focused approach in your work the more you learn to believe and trust in your clients; it enables you to see that the clients and/or carers can determine for themselves what is, or is not, possible. One successful outcome can be enough to dispel the fear of asking a future-oriented question with clients who have a progressive disease or terminal diagnosis. If it works, do more of it.

Key points

- SFBT is best learnt through an experiential approach
- Trust your clients – they will find solutions
- The practitioner aims to help clients discover their best hopes for the future

Summary

Whether it is for a single session or as part of a number of sessions, SFBT is being used successfully in the group setting. It can be incorporated into an existing framework that is largely educational in nature, and an example is given to show how this can be done gradually over a period of time. It can also be used in conjunction with other therapeutic techniques; solution focused questions can provide a group with an activity or game to start the session, and miracle questions/scales can help elicit individual client goals. Staff training/development can also benefit from these techniques. Training sessions often promote discussion about change within the workplace and some commonly asked questions were explored in this chapter.

Chapter 8
Solutions in care aims

Many therapists and other health professionals can develop a sense of burnout; a feeling that they are not managing their caseload effectively or accomplishing what they learnt at college. There is the perception that the focus on evidence based practice puts further pressure on the professional, rather than facilitating the reflective process on the desired outcome with the patient. A useful way to evaluate clinical effectiveness is the Malcomess care aims model, which describes and measures the

> clinical reasoning and decision-making involved in good practice ... Unlike diagnostically driven care, it suggests that effective care focuses on reducing the risk and impact of a presenting problem, not necessarily reducing or resolving the problem. (Malcomess, 2001)

The SLT department at the Chelsea and Westminster Hospital has been using this model since 2001. The case examples discussed in this chapter aim to show how it has helped clinical work with a variety of client groups, with particular reference given to how SFBT has been part of this move away from a diagnosis-centred to a more client-centred agenda. Outcomes from two audits carried out during this time will be discussed, as well as outcomes and references specifically related to research on SFBT.

Overview of the model

The Malcomess care aims work in agreed episodes of care using measurable goals to evaluate outcome of care after each episode. To identify their focus for a particular period of care therapists use one of eight different care aims: Assessment, Maintenance, Anticipatory, Supportive, Palliative, Enabling, Curative and Rehabilitation. Care aims can be used with any client group as, like SFBT, the focus is on reducing the risk or impact of a problem. It may not be possible to reduce or resolve the problem itself. All intervention must aim to reduce risk to the client first whether it is psychological, functional or physical so that the higher the risk the shorter the episode. The care aim is determined by what the client or carer want to be different and the resources the professional can offer to help achieve their goals and/or reduce their risk.

Kate Malcomess is keen to emphasize that using care aims is more about understanding a process rather than undertaking a paper-filling exercise. Training is needed to use care aims effectively, and literature is available for further information on the model (Anderson and Van der Gaag, 2005). The form given here is one that has been developed at the Chelsea and Westminster Hospital to include the core elements: type of care aim, level of input, episode goal, evidence, sub goals and predicted length of episode/ number of sessions. Data is documented alongside this for outcome measures.

Working with care aims and SFBT

Individuality

There are a number of similarities in the thinking behind care aims and SFBT. Most important is the recognition that clients cannot be put into exact categories. Looking at a medical classification of diagnoses alone tends to focus you on the physical risk rather than the functional or psychological impact of a disease.

> Studies show that diagnosis alone does not predict service needs, length of hospitalization, level of care or functional outcomes. Nor is the presence of a disease or disorder an accurate predictor of receipt of disability benefits, work performance, return to work potential, or likelihood of social integration. (WHO, 2002)

Impact

In addition to impairment work students need to be trained in clinical reasoning and process, so that the focus moves away from simply analysing the 'foot problem' or 'speech problem' to noticing the impact of that problem on the clients lives and what the professional can, realistically, do about it.

An example is useful here. An SLT may do some impairment work on language which involves facilitating clients in categorization skills. What evidence is there that this will make a difference to the clients or contribute to a better quality of life? Clients can learn better categorization skills in clinic, but there may be no perceived change in the clients' episode goal that 'they will be more able to select items from the hospital menu'. Reflective practice and working within episodes of care means that therapy goals are constantly reviewed and that effectiveness is measured. SFBT can provide individualized rating scales that can facilitate this process of measuring the focus of care rather than whether the condition has changed.

Client goals

Action plans and tasks tend to describe what therapists are doing to clients. Care aims are concerned with goals and *why* therapists are involved with a client at a particular time. This makes them

> more client-focused as it helps them recognize the centrality of the client's views, attitudes and motivation to the effectiveness of their care and it supports them in determining which clients are most likely to benefit from their care. (Malcomess, 2001)

Creating goals with clients can be difficult as they often have clear ideas about the problem rather than the steps they could take towards resolving them. Furthermore clients change and they may have shifting goals that reflect the current focus in their lives, making it difficult to commit goals to paper. SFBT allows you to constantly refocus on goals and to ensure that they are positive, as specific as possible and are written in the clients' language.

Key points

- Always remember that every case is different
- Use goals to measure effectiveness
- Keep it client-focused.

A care aim measures the outcome of the episode goal rather than the outcome of each sub goal. The importance of this is demonstrated in the following case examples.

Case example

Client: I find it difficult to control my temper and I get stressed. I was planning to go and visit my son in Australia, and now I don't know if I can.

The SLT is asked to do a bedside assessment of this client's communication following a stroke. Although it is immediately apparent that there are no difficulties with speech or language it is clear that the client is having some difficulty dealing with his emotions about his present condition. The therapist decides that the clinical risk is psychological and that the care aim is Supportive rather than simply one of Assessment. Using a solution focused approach they discuss times when the client is communicating his feelings more effectively, and by the end of the session he reports he is feeling less distressed. The SLT alerts the stroke team to the psychological risk and concludes that the episode goal ('Mr A will be calmer during the session') has had a successful outcome. He is discharged from speech and language therapy.

There is often the complaint that the role of the therapist in the acute setting is only one of assessment. However, care aims can give a more accurate picture; once you start treating then Assessment is no longer the care aim but becomes a sub goal within the care aim, which in this case is Supportive. This is a better description of the particular requirements of both the client and the therapist, providing feedback about the different factors affecting service delivery.

The client is re-admitted to hospital a month later with further difficulties and the SLT opens a new episode. The risk that his eating and drinking may be compromised requires the focus of care to be an assessment of his swallow.

Case example

Ahmed is 24 and has a severe stammer. His self rating on the WASSP shows 'very severe' ratings across most of the parameters (Figure 8.1) indicating difficulties with body structure and function, activity/participation and contextual factors. Using the miracle question and scales he identifies his episode goal as the ability to feel more confident about his speech. In the first session he rates his feelings about his communication as fluctuating between 2 and 5, and he would like this to become more stable.

The therapist uses her knowledge of working with SFBT and people who stammer to predict that change in attitude or feelings can take place within four sessions. In fact Ahmed begins to notice he is more 'calmed down' after two sessions and decides he would like to 'talk with people more'. The episode goal changes and the focus of care is on use of function; the care aim becomes Enabling.

This is part of the final session:

Therapist:	What has been working well since I last saw you?
Ahmed:	I went to my country. My talking was better with my father. I was calm. I was able to talk to more people and it was easier.
Therapist:	What was different about talking with your father? That was important for you, wasn't it?
Ahmed:	Yes. Very important. It was not like father/son. It was like a friend of mine. My system was calmed down. He noticed, and so did other people.
Therapist:	What do you need to do to keep it going?
Ahmed:	I have to trust that person as my friend. I don't have to think about my speaking. I have to trust in myself.
Therapist:	You have to believe in yourself more.

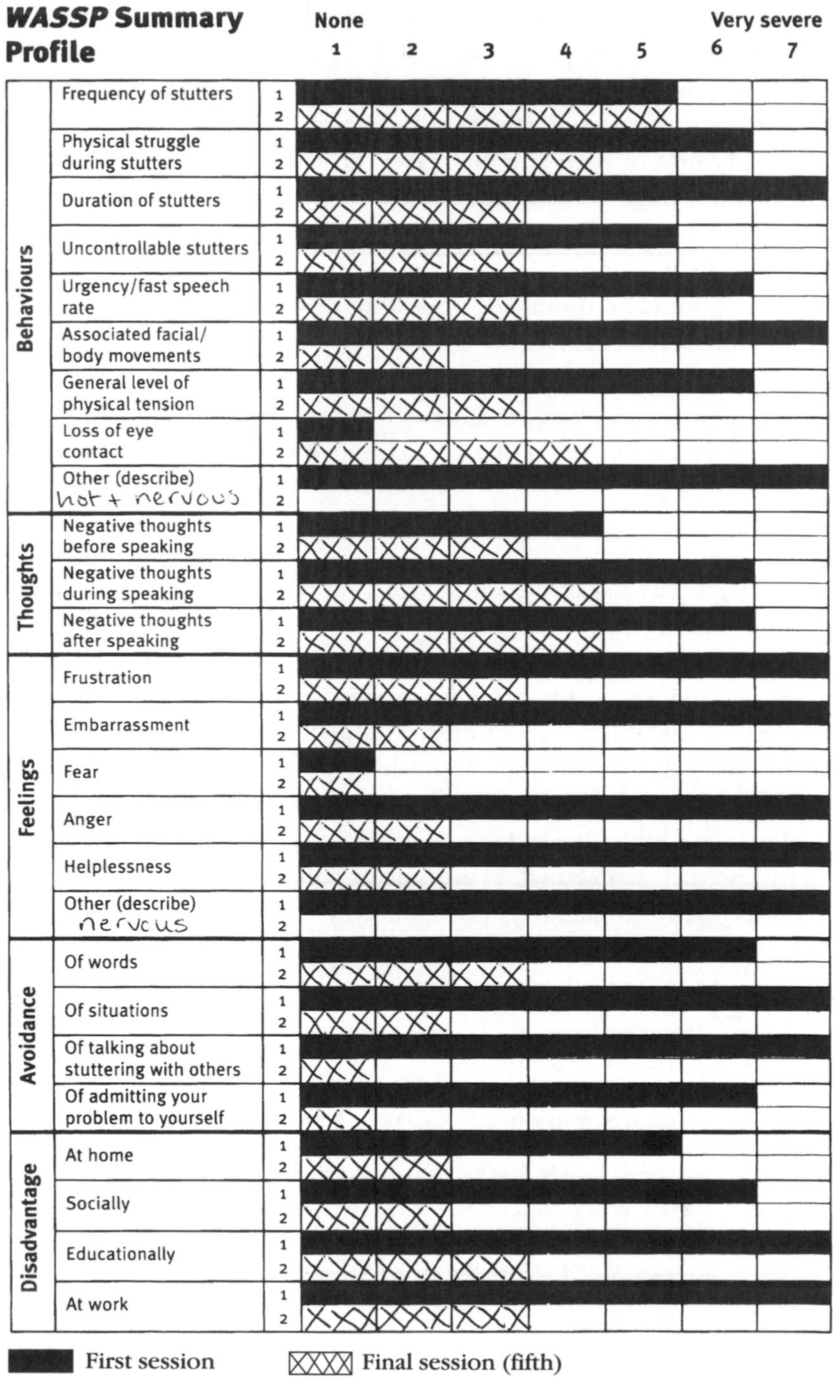

WASSP Summary Profile

Scale: None (1) 2 3 4 5 6 7 (Very severe)

Each item is rated over two sessions: row 1 = First session (■ solid bar), row 2 = Final session (fifth) (XXXX).

Behaviours
- Frequency of stutters
- Physical struggle during stutters
- Duration of stutters
- Uncontrollable stutters
- Urgency/fast speech rate
- Associated facial/body movements
- General level of physical tension
- Loss of eye contact
- Other (describe) hot + nervous

Thoughts
- Negative thoughts before speaking
- Negative thoughts during speaking
- Negative thoughts after speaking

Feelings
- Frustration
- Embarrassment
- Fear
- Anger
- Helplessness
- Other (describe) nervous

Avoidance
- Of words
- Of situations
- Of talking about stuttering with others
- Of admitting your problem to yourself

Disadvantage
- At home
- Socially
- Educationally
- At work

Legend: ■ First session   XXXX Final session (fifth)

Figure 8.1 Ahmed. Reproduced with permission from WASSP: Wright & Ayre Stuttering Self-Rating Profile, Louise Wright and Anne Ayre, Speechmark Publishing/Winslow Press, Bicester, 2000.

Ahmed: Yes. I have to think about that. Last night I was with my friends in a pub. I was talking not very well but I felt it was good. I was talking with a girl for four hours! First I was too shy, but after one hour I was calmed down. I was talking with her with my mind. I have to keep myself more relaxed.

The therapist feels it is a good moment to look at the WASSP again and Ahmed is pleased when he compares the original scores with his current rating.

Ahmed: God gave me a good mind. I have my skills and I have to use them.
Therapist: How has this session been useful?
Ahmed: You give me some power. I don't worry, I talk with people. I feel confident. I don't think about before – bad speaker – but look for now and in front of me.

Ahmed is encouraged to contact the department again in the future if he requires further assistance. Both the therapist and client feel they have achieved two successful outcomes from five sessions over a period of five months (Figures 8.2 and 8.3). The care aims highlight evidence to support this assumption, but there are also two sessions which have been videoed (session three and session five). These show a change in Ahmed's speech which is realistically portrayed in his summary of behaviours, with the exception that there is improvement (rather than deterioration as he sees it) in eye contact.

At no time in the sessions does the therapist focus on specific techniques to help with the stammer. Handouts are given to Ahmed at the end of the first session regarding breathing techniques that he says he will read at home, and information is also given on groups and contacts with other people who stammer but Ahmed does not pursue these avenues.

Key point

- SFBT can help reduce the risk or impact of a problem whether it is psychological, functional or physical.

Monitoring mechanism

A SFBT practitioner knows that, regardless of the particular client group, the basic techniques help to identify an awareness that change is happening, and to explore concrete ways for change to occur in the future. Miracle questions promote the development of appropriately designed goals and exception questions focus on developing solutions. Coping and scaling questions quantify clients' thoughts, clarify the steps needed to reach their

CHELSEA & WESTMINSTER HEALTHCARE NHS TRUST
SPEECH & LANGUAGE THERAPY DEPARTMENT

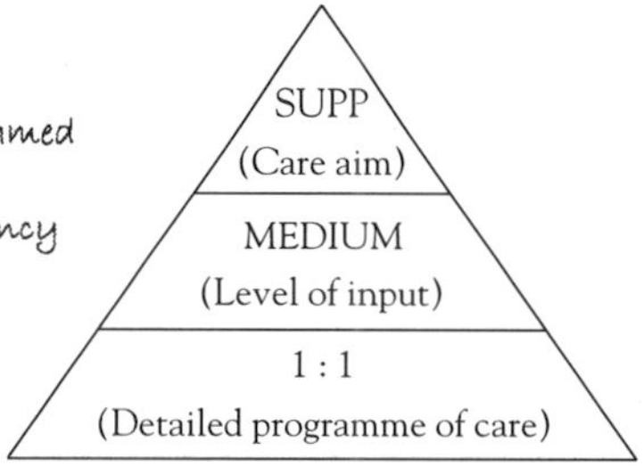

CARE AIM

Patient's Name: *Ahmed*
d.o.b.
Diagnosis: *Dysfluency*
SLT:

SUPP (Care aim)
MEDIUM (Level of input)
1 : 1
(Detailed programme of care)

Dysphagia ☐ Communication ☐ Voice ☐ Dysfluency ☑

Status: New Referral ☑ (1) Existing Client ☐ (2)

State actual length of episode of care in sessions:

1☐ 2☑ 3☐ 4☐ 5☐ 6☐ 7☐ 8☐ 9☐ 10☐ 11☐ 12☐ 13☐ 14☐ 15☐ 16☐
17☐ 18☐ 19☐ 20☐ 21☐ 22☐ 23☐ 24☐ sessions

DATE OF COMMENCEMENT OF EPISODE ...../...../.....

DATE OF COMPLETION OF EPISODE ...../...../.....

Result of this episode?
Outcome achieved ☑ (1)
Outcome not achieved ☐ (2)
Episode incomplete ☐ (3)

Reason..

Next step: Discharge ☐ (1)
Further S&L input inappropriate ☐ (2)
Further episode opened ☑ (3)
Transfer ☐ (4)
Waiting list ☐ (5)

Parent/Carer Signature....................... date...........

Therapist Signature....................... date...........

Episode Goal:
Ahmed will feel more confident about his speech

Evidence:
There will be less fluctuation between 2–5 on self rating scale

Sub Goals:
1. *Ahmed will notice the times when he is communicating and "calmed down"*
2. *Ahmed will identify what he is doing at these times to help with communication*
3. *Ahmed will receive information from the SLT re possible exercises and courses to help with dysfluency*
4.

Predicted number of sessions: *4*

Predicted length of episode:

Figure 8.2 Ahmed: first care aim (sessions 1 and 2)

CHELSEA & WESTMINSTER HEALTHCARE NHS TRUST
SPEECH & LANGUAGE THERAPY DEPARTMENT

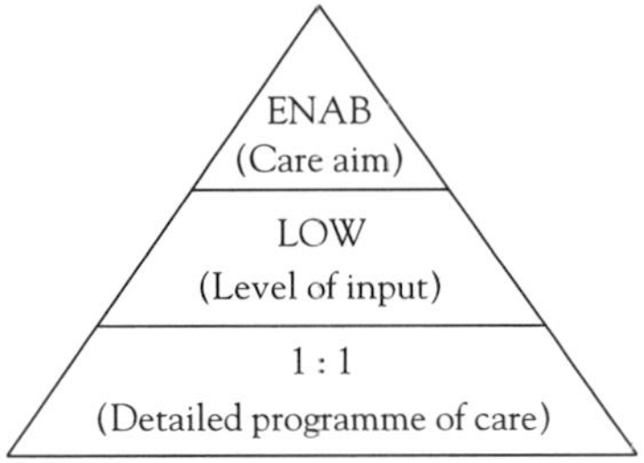

Dysphagia ☐   **Communication** ☐   **Voice** ☐   **Dysfluency** ☑

Status: **New Referral** ☐ (1)   **Existing Client** ☑ (2)

State actual length of episode of care in sessions:

1☐ 2☐ 3☑ 4☐ 5☐ 6☐ 7☐ 8☐ 9☐ 10☐ 11☐ 12☐ 13☐ 14☐ 15☐ 16☐

17☐ 18☐ 19☐ 20☐ 21☐ 22☐ 23☐ 24☐ **sessions**

DATE OF COMMENCEMENT OF EPISODE ...../...../......

DATE OF COMPLETION OF EPISODE ...../...../......

Result of this episode?   Outcome achieved   (1) ☑
   Outcome not achieved   (2) ☐
   Episode incomplete   (3) ☐

Reason...

Next step: Discharge   (1) ☑
   Further S&L input inappropriate   (2) ☐
   Further episode opened   (3) ☐
   Transfer   (4) ☐
   Waiting list   (5) ☐

Parent/Carer Signature................................ date................

Therapist Signature................................ date................

CARE AIM

Patient's Name: Ahmed

d.o.b.

Diagnosis: Dysfluency

SLT:

ENAB
(Care aim)

LOW
(Level of input)

1 : 1

(Detailed programme of care)

Episode Goal:
Ahmed will be talking with people more

Evidence:
WASSP

Sub Goals:
1. Ahmed will be talking more with friends

2. Ahmed will be talking more with others

3. Ahmed "won't have to think about" his speaking

4.

Predicted number of sessions: 4

Predicted length of episode:

Figure 8.3 Ahmed: second care aim (sessions 3, 4, 5)

goals and assess progress. Based on outcome studies on SFBT and their own experience, practitioners are not surprised that successful outcomes occur within a relatively short period of time.

Care aims enable practitioners to monitor the caseload in a more detailed fashion. It does not mean that they will hypothesize that all clients who stammer, for example, will need a Supportive care aim. However, care aims can demonstrate that, using the SFBT approach, practitioners can help the client feel differently about their condition (Supportive), help the client manage their condition and/or use their existing function more or in different ways (Enabling), or facilitate lasting change in their condition (Curative/Rehabilitation). Using the care aim form, practitioners can look back over their caseload and give a precise account of episode goals and sub goals as discussed with the client. They can show that they are able 'to predict outcomes and reflect regularly on their practice – the cornerstones of evidence-based practice' (Malcomess, 2001).

As part of this reflective process an SLT took a sample of her caseload over the previous 18 months when care aims have been used. The clients selected are five males and two females between the ages of 23 and 34. Six of the clients have been referred for help with their stammer and a further client is diagnosed as having 'speech dyspraxia'. SFBT is the approach used throughout the sessions, while handouts are given on further information (groups and the British Stammering Association) and specific techniques (usually breathing) at the end of the session.

The following observations are made:

1. Four males feel they need to feel more relaxed and confident about their speech and the care aim is Supportive. Their self-rating scales about their speech vary from 1 – 8, which bear no relation to the outward severity of the stammer. The client who gives his level as 1 is asked coping questions to help him identify how he has been managing in difficult circumstances. The client who is at 8 explores the 10% difference (he is a mathematician!) that he feels is so important to his functioning. Both come for two sessions and are then discharged.

The other two clients (at 5 and 6/7) only come for one session. When asked how the session has been useful their comments are as follows:

Client: Maybe I could think about the language less. I find this scaling question useful. It gives me more confidence.

Client: I feel I'm addressing it. Coming here was a big thing – my girlfriend has been nagging me. It's about talking to someone who knows about stammering.

2. Two clients, at 2 and 4.5 on their scales, feel they are able to effect change in their work environments. The care aim is Enabling, and SFBT helps them to establish the framework to notice change in their functional ability. The female and male client come for two and three sessions respectively and achieve their episode goal, although not all the strategies that they develop are listed in their sub goals:

Client: (*goal is to use the telephone more*) I've done some more phone calls. I've discovered that if I say 'I'm not very good on the phone' it's much better. But my life is generally better. I think I really need to start feeling more security in my life and start sorting out my cash!

Client: (*goal is to be more verbal at college*) I've asked out my group twice for a beer! I'm saying more. I went for an interview last week and I began by saying, 'If I stammer, bear with me. I stammer in stressful situations but it's not normally a big issue with me.' I've never said that before. Didn't plan to do it but it definitely helped. I left the interview, and for the first time felt that I've said all the things I wanted to say.

The WASSP rating sheet shows changes for this second client over three sessions across all five sub-scales that address the overt, covert and social dimensions of stammering. SFBT can effect change in emotions and feelings whether or not this is the focus of therapy, just as a focus on activity and participation can also have a knock-on effect on stammering behaviours. There is food for thought here as to service provision for clients who stammer.

3. The last client in this study, referred with 'speech dyspraxia', is a 23-year-old female who says she used to have a stammer. In two sessions she moves from 4/5 to 7/8. There is little evidence of difficulty in her speech, and the SLT feels she can facilitate lasting change in the client's condition. The care aim is, therefore, Rehabilitation, although an alternative label in this context could be Improvement.

The first session involves the miracle question, looking at exceptions and scales. The second session identifies the times when things have been working well since she was first seen two weeks previously:

Client: I've been talking and initiating a lot more. People understand me more. Everything's falling into place.

Therapist: How have you managed to do that?

Client: I've been trying to make the effort with other people. I realize it's a skill rather than being innate – you can become a good communicator by learning social skills.

Therapist:	I was impressed in the last session that you have 9/10 confidence you will achieve your goal. Have you always been a determined person?
Client:	Stupid, yes! Now I'll have an opportunity to try out my skills in presentations at college. I know if I don't do one well it's not the end of the world.
Therapist:	You've got the right language. Opportunity rather than challenge!

Key point

■   At the time of discharge six of the seven clients were at 5 or above on their scales.

Care aims in a group setting

The group at the Chelsea and Westminster Hospital for outpatients who have dysphasia has already been described in Chapter 7. Ana, Richard, James and Alan all have case notes which detail the weekly session plan and outcome, but the care aim is a useful reminder that there is an overriding episode goal that may differ for each group member.

There is no such thing as a team care aim. In the case of this particular group there is a goal for the group, which is that the SLT will provide a supportive environment to work on functional communication. The care aims, however, look at the impact of the stroke on each group member, and this helps maintain a focus on therapy given to each individual rather than a blanket provision of therapy for clients with varying needs. They also help identify evidence that therapy has been effective for each client, which is almost impossible to do at a collective group level.

The SLT identifies Ana's highest level of risk as being psychological and aims to facilitate change in how she feels about her condition (Supportive). Her episode goal is as follows:

Ana:	She will feel more confident as she experiences successful communication in the group.

The SLT feels that she may not be able to facilitate lasting change in Richard's, James's or Alan's condition (Curative/Rehabilitation) but that she can help them use their existing function more or in different ways (Enabling). However, each client has an episode goal which is most pertinent to that individual:

Richard:	He will be more competent at expressing himself to others both inside and outside the group.

James: He will be able to communicate more effectively with others both
                  inside and outside the group.

Alan: He will develop gesture and verbal description skills to compensate
                  for word-finding difficulties and dyspraxic-like features in his
                  speech.

Evidence and sub-goals will differ. What is important is the reflective process
involved in determining (a) whether attending the group can effect change
and (b) the recognition that goals must be reviewed regularly. If the SLT gets
her hypothesis wrong and the care aim needs to be changed then this
demonstrates good clinical decision-making rather than poor therapy. Care
aims support collaborative working with the client in a way that is sensitive
to the clients' needs and what the therapist is able to provide.

Key points

■   'Collaborative working', 'measurable goals', 'inclusive of all clients' and
     'regular review' are all phrases that occur in effective clinical governance
     systems. The Malcomess care aims and SBT work well together to provide a
     framework to promote good evidence-based practice.

Evidence

It can be difficult to prove that change has occurred as a result of therapy,
particularly if there is spontaneous recovery after a neurological event. It is
therefore necessary to establish a baseline, and predict that within x number
of sessions/weeks/months change will occur to a given point. At the end of
an episode, it is decided whether the outcome has been achieved or not.

The WASSP, which is both an assessment and outcome measure, identifies
the need to examine not only body structure and function but also the
activity, participation and attitudinal aspects of a client. It has the advantage
of being quick and easy to administer. However, there is a need for similar
material with other client groups, especially when it comes to measuring
change in the perception of well-being. Studies on the level of SLT reliability
using the Therapy Outcome Measure (TOM) show the need for sufficient
training and practice opportunities to achieve an acceptable level of
reliability, particularly when measuring the psychosocial domains of
handicap/social participation and well-being (John and Enderby, 2000).
Increasingly, quality of life is becoming popular for use as an outcome
measure but there needs to be the recognition that this is individualistic. 'It is
unrealistic to assume that one person's perception of what constitutes a
good quality of life is the same as another's' (Power, 2003).

The advantage of a continuous line rating scales from 0 to 10, without intermediate scores, is that they can be sensitive to very small changes, and progress can be measured not only in terms of gains achieved but also by looking at the percentage of goals achieved. The value of goal attainment scaling is that it can measure change that is valued by the patient and there is evidence that 'even the more severely cognitive impaired participants can participate in goal selection' (Malec, 1999).

Applying the points in this discussion to how evidence is used in care aims it may be useful to look at a specific example. There may be occasions when an SLT will need to explore non-speech modes as augmentative and/or alternative means of communication. A client learns how to operate a switch on a piece of equipment: the clients' goal is that this will enable him to communicate more with others and the evidence is a measurement of change in this context. Evidence is not a measurement of how effective he is at operating the switch, although this will be documented by the SLT. The care aim ensures that the focus of therapy is on changing the impact of the condition on a clients' life (i.e. *why* you are doing therapy) rather than a description of what you, the therapist, are doing. It is focused on client goals rather than therapy tasks, and data collection becomes an integral part of clinical care using the reflective loop when deciding to open an episode. It brings together efficacy and effectiveness.

The problem, of course, with measuring behaviours on scales that are of specific value to the patient is that they can only be used as before and after measures of change for one client. You can show clinical effectiveness, but it is another story if what is required is efficacy in highly controlled settings. It has been suggested that studies

> can include a combination of features of efficacy and effectiveness studies ... [and] that highly controlled efficacy studies may not be feasible or even possible in service delivery settings, and if they are, they may be sufficiently lacking in clinical validity as to be of questionable use. (Gingerich and Eisengart, 2000)

Key point

■   SFBT and care aims focus on client goals rather than therapy tasks

---

Outcome studies on SFBT/research

A large study was carried out at the Brief Family Therapy Center (BFTC) from November 1992 to August 1993 on 275 of their clients. SFBT was found to be effective with a diversity of clients, with the same therapeutic procedures being effective across a range of problems identified by the clients. More than three-quarters of the clients either fully met their treatment goals or made progress towards them, and this level of effectiveness occurred over an average of 2.9 sessions. Outcomes were measured using scaling questions and contact with the client seven to nine months after their final sessions (Miller et al., 1996).

This data suggests positive outcomes, wide applicability across diverse client groups and a lower average number of sessions compared to other more established approaches. Other outcome studies at the BFTC show similar results and help increase the credibility of SFBT. There are also process studies that have examined the immediate or long-term impact of a particular therapeutic intervention or strategy; pre-treatment change, solution talk and homework tasks between the first and second session are just some of the examples of SFBT interventions that have been explored. Examples of these studies are given by A. Jay McKeel, who suggests that in the past 'researchers have relied too much on "objective" measure and ratings by therapists and/or outside observers. Clinicians want to know what clients find useful about treatment' (Miller et al., 1996).

Gingerich and Eisengart (2000) provide a review of all the controlled studies of SFBT client outcomes appearing in the English literature up to and including 1999. Client outcomes are taken to be client behaviour or function rather than client satisfaction, and the intervention has to include one or more of the following core components:

1. a search for pre-session change
2. goal-setting
3. use of the miracle question
4. use of scaling questions
5. a search for exceptions
6. a consultation break
7. a message including compliments and task (Gingerich and Eisengart, 2000).

One study, considered well-controlled, is undertaken by Cockburn et al. (1997): 'Solution-focused therapy and psychosocial adjustment to orthopaedic rehabilitation in a work hardening program'. The patients receive either the standard rehabilitation protocol or SFBT (once a week for one hour during a six-week period), and results show that the SFBT groups have significantly better social supports and psychosocial adjustments than patients in the control group. The authors add:

> The most encouraging outcome was reflected in the work re-entry rates for those patients participating in the treatment group with 68% returning in less than 7 days after discharge as opposed to approximately 4% of the control group. (Cockburn et al., 1997)

Although their study does not use a randomized design, Zimmerman et al. (1997) also found significant results when using SFBT on couples (who met weekly over a period of six weeks) to help improve marital satisfaction. The Dyadic Adjustment Scale (DAS) scores for the treatment group revealed statistically significant improvement on the total score and all four subscale scores. Indeed, post-test scores for the treatment group had improved to levels approaching the pretest scores of the nondistressed control group.

Care pathways

Once data is collated you can start tracking care pathways for individual clients. While a SFBT practitioner would not advocate standardizing care pathways for particular client groups, it is important to be aware of the difference the approach can make when predicting episode length. Furthermore, 'most services which have adopted the care aims approach have reported a significant increase in the level of discharge' (Malcomess, 2001).

Care aims can make you more aware of when an outcome has been unsuccessful. An example is a man whose episode goal is 'to be communicating more effectively on the ward'. Evidence of this is that the intelligibility of his speech will have increased from single-syllable to three-syllable words. There is no change in his communication at the end of the episode and the SLT is forced to explore other possibilities. On reflection it appears that he does not achieve carryover from therapy input and the SLT feels she is unable to effect change in attitude, function or condition. He is discharged.

A different picture emerges with David, who is also admitted to hospital with a stroke. He has a similar episode goal to the previous man but, although he is initially somewhat confused, he does not appear to have any cognitive impairment. A bedside assessment is carried out on his communication, but the main thrust of input is to effect immediate change in his condition. The first care aim is therefore Rehabilitation, which is then followed by Assessment, as he is no longer confused and a more detailed profile of his communication is needed by the stroke team, the SLT and David himself.

David has been in hospital for nearly seven weeks. He has become increasingly labile and anxious about his condition, making effective participation in therapy with the stroke team more difficult.

David: I'll never be able to play the piano again. David is dead. I know
            there is no memory after death, but this is death with a memory.

He is seen by a psychiatric nurse, but both he and his family are adamant that there should be no further medication. The SLT feels the clinical risk to David is psychological and opens an episode that is focused on boosting his sense of dignity and self-esteem, incorporating SFBT techniques (miracle question, looking for exceptions and scales) into the session alongside some communication work. Although David is aware that he is emotionally labile because of his current condition, he is keen to reduce the amount of crying that occurs when he communicates with others. The SLT sees David for six sessions over a period of four weeks (low input) and keeps in close contact with his family. This Supportive care aim is completed prior to his discharge home where he awaits admission into an intensive rehabilitation centre.

The information shown in David's care pathway (Figure 8.4) is easily accessible from his three existing care aims. Even if you are not an SLT you can develop a greater understanding of the thinking process into her delivery of care than a treatment plan can ever divulge. She has been able to predict outcomes accurately over a period of time from referral to discharge and gives this information in a succinct fashion without, you will note, referring to a detailed description of diagnosis. The care aims framework has facilitated her decision making process and SFBT has been an essential part of her repertoire of skills.

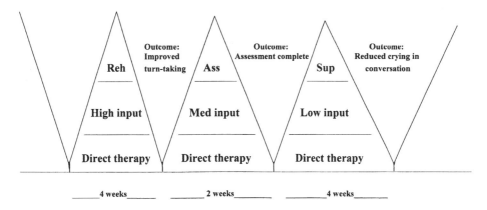

Figure 8.4 65 year old man – labile following a stroke, SLT

An audit of care aims at the Chelsea and Westminster Hospital from July 2001 to September 2002 shows that the overall success rate is 83 per cent. Another audit on outpatients from October 2002 to December 2003 gives the overall success rate as 94 per cent, more than half of these care aims being Rehabilitation and Assessment, followed by Supportive. Eighty-two per cent of the outpatients are being treated within four sessions.

Summary

Both SFBT and care aims recognize the importance of client goals and the belief that it is the practitioners' job to reduce the impact of the problem rather than looking at a medical classification of diagnosis alone. By looking at the preferred future, SFBT can provide the episode goal within a care aim, and the evidence that it has been achieved is elicited through exceptions and scaling questions. Throughout the book examples are given to show effectiveness within the group setting and on an individual basis where SFBT has determined change in the function, activity, participation and attitudinal aspects of a client. Outcome studies on SFBT and research demonstrate that these findings are becoming increasingly widespread.

It is hoped that this book has provided information that will allow the reader to embark on the solution focused journey with confidence and that the case histories have shown the range and diversity of SFBT in its application to our clients. There is a growing awareness of this approach, and positive outcomes in our clinical practice offer a robust case for using SFBT more widely in the hospital and community setting.

References

Anderson C, Van der Gaag A (eds) (2005) Speech and Language Therapy: Issues in Professional Practice. London: Whurr Publishers.

Berg IK (1991, revised 1999) Family Preservation: A Brief Therapy Workbook. London: Brief Therapy Press.

Berg IK (2000) Working Briefly. London: BRIEF.

Berg IK, Jick K (1995) Making Home Visits. Brief Family Therapy Center.

Berg IK, Reuss N (1998) Solutions Step by Step: A Substance Abuse Treatment Manual. New York: Norton & Wylie.

Bowles N, Mackintosh C, Torn A (2001) Nurses' communication skills: an evaluation of the impact of solution-focused communication training. Journal of Advanced Nursing 36(3): 347-54.

Brajtman S, Azoulay D, Gassner R, Yeheskel M (2002) Malignant brain tumours and palliative care. European Journal of Palliative Care 9(1).

Bray D (2003) Presentation on SFBT. London: The Royal Marsden.

Brimblecombe N (1995) The use of brief therapy as part of the nursing care plan. Nursing Times 91(35).

Brumfitt S (1998) The measurement of psychological well-being in the person with aphasia. International Journal of Language & Communication Disorders 33, supplement: 116-20.

Brumfitt S (2003) Psychosocial Aspects; Signposts to the Future. British Aphasiology Society Biennial Conference.

Brumfitt S, Sheeran P (1999) VASES: Visual Analogue Self-Esteem Scale. Bicester: Winslow Press.

Burns K (1999) Focusing on success: brief therapy in practice. RCSLT Bulletin, November: 10-11.

Cade B, O'Hanlon B (1993) A Brief Guide to Brief Therapy. New York: Norton.

Cockburn JT, Thomas FN, Cockburn OJ (1997) Solution-focused therapy and psychosocial adjustment to orthopaedic rehabilitation in a work hardening program. Journal of Occupational Rehabilitation 7(2): 97-106.

Cream A, Onslow M, Packman A, Llewellyn G (2003) Protection from harm: the experience of adults after therapy with prolonged-speech. International Journal of Language & Communication Disorders 38(4): 379-95

De Jong P, Berg IK (2002) Interviewing for Solutions. Pacific Grove, CA: Brooks/Cole.

de Shazer S (1988) Clues: Investigating Solutions in Brief Therapy. New York: Norton.

de Shazer S, Dolan Y, Berg IK (2004) Taking Emotions Seriously. Amsterdam: EBTA Conference.

Dolan Y (2000) Beyond Survival. London: Brief Therapy Press.

George E (2003) Beyond Solutions. Berlin: EBTA Conference.

George E, Iveson C, Ratner H (1990, revised/expanded 1999) Problem to Solution: Brief Therapy with Individuals and Families. London: Brief Therapy Press.

George E, Iveson C, Ratner H (2003) Solution Focused Brief Therapy: Course Notes. London: BRIEF.

Gingerich W, Eisengart S (2000) Solution-focused brief therapy: a review of the outcome research. Family Process 39(4): 477-98.

Hayhow R, Levy C (1989) Working with Stuttering. Bicester: Winslow Press.

Iveson C (1994) Solution Focused Brief Therapy: establishing goals and assessing competence. British Journal of Occupational Therapy 57(3): 95-8.

Iveson C (2001) Whose Life? Working with Older People. London: Brief Therapy Press.

Iveson C (2002) Solution-focused brief therapy. Advances in Psychiatric Treatment 8: 149-56.

Jackson PZ, McKergow M (2002) The Solutions Focus. The SIMPLE way to positive change. London: Nicholas Brealey Publishing.

John A, Enderby P (2000) Reliability of speech and language therapists using therapy outcome measures. International Journal of Language and Communication Disorders 35(2): 287-302.

Kelson M, Riesel J, Kennelly C (2001) Speaking Out about Stroke Services. The views of people affected by stroke: a survey to inform the implementation of the National Service Framework for Older People. The Stroke Association.

LaPointe L (1999) Quality of life with aphasia. Seminars in Speech and Language 20(1): 5-15.

Lee M-Y (1997) A study of solution-focused brief therapy: outcomes and issues. American Journal of Family Therapy 25: 3-17.

Lock S, Wilkinson R, Bryan K (2001) SPPARC – Supporting Partners of People with Aphasia in Relationships and Conversation. Speechmark Publishing Ltd.

McClenahan R, Weinman J (1998) Determinants of carer distress in non-acute stroke. International Journal of Language & Communication Disorders 33, supplement: 138-42.

Macdonald A (2004) Solution Focused Practice: Existing Competencies and Preferred Futures. Preston: UKASP Conference.

McKergow M (ed.) (2003) Positive Approaches to Change. Organisations & People 10(4).

McNally R, Bryant R, Ehlers A (2003) Does early psychological intervention promote recovery from posttraumatic stress? American Psychological Society 4(2): 45-79.

Malcomess K (2001) The reason for care. RCSLT Bulletin, November.

Malec J (1999) Goal attainment scaling in rehabilitation. Neuropsychological Rehabilitation 9(3/4): 253-75.

Martin S, Darnley L (2004) The Teaching Voice, 2nd edn. London: Whurr Publishers.

Metcalf L (1998) Solution Focused Group Therapy. New York: Simon & Schuster.

Miller S, Hubble M, Duncan B (eds) (1996) Handbook of Solution-Focused Brief Therapy. San Francisco, CA: Jossey-Bass.

O'Connell B, Palmer S (eds) (2003) Handbook of Solution-Focused Therapy. London: Sage.

O'Hanlon B, Beadle S (1996) A Field Guide to Possibility Land. London: Brief Therapy Press.

Power T (2003) Outcome Measurement in Neurology. Therapy Weekly 30(25): 7-10.

Ratner H (1999) Staying Brief: A Follow-up Course in Solution Focused Brief Therapy. London: BRIEF.

Sharry J (2001) Solution-focused Groupwork. London: Sage.

Sharry J, Madden B, Darmody M (2001) Becoming a Solution Detective: A Strengths-based Guide to Brief Therapy. London: Brief Therapy Press.

Solution Focused Therapy listserv (SFT-L) 4 April 2003.

Swinburn K, Morley R (1996) Parkinson's Disease Management Pack. London: Whurr Publishers.

Thompson R, Littrell JM (1998) Brief counseling for students with learning disabilities. Professional School Counseling 2(1): 60–7.

Vaughn K, Hastings-Guerrero S, Kassner C (1996) Solution-oriented inpatient group therapy. Journal of Systemic Therapies 15(3): 1–13.

Wales P (1998) Solution-focused brief therapy in primary care. Nursing Times 94 (15).

Walter J, Peller J (1992) Becoming Solution Focused in Brief Therapy. New York: Brunner/Mazel.

Weiner-Davis M (1992) Divorce Busting: A Revolutionary and Rapid Program for Staying Together. New York: Simon & Schuster.

White M (1995) Re-Authoring Lives: Interviews and Essays. Adelaide: Dulwich Centre Publications.

Winbolt B (2002) Accentuate the positive. Therapy Weekly 28(43).

World Health Organization (2001) Disability and Rehabilitation Team. Rethinking Care. Geneva: WHO.

World Health Organization (2002) Towards a Common Language for Functioning, Disability and Health. Geneva: WHO.

Wright L, Ayre A (2000) WASSP: The Wright & Ayre Stuttering Self-Rating Profile. Bicester: Winslow Press Ltd.

Ylvisaker M, Feeney T (2000) Reconstruction of identity after traumatic brain injury. Brain Impairment 1: 12–28.

Ylvisaker M, Feeney J, Feeney T (1999) An everyday approach to long-term rehabilitation after traumatic brain injury. Cornett B (ed.) Clinical Practice Management in Speech-Language Pathology: Principles and Practicalities 117–62. Gaithersburg, MD: Aspen Publishing Co.

Ylvisaker M, Jacobs H, Feeney T (2003) Positive supports for people who experience behavioral and cognitive disability after brain injury. Journal Head Trauma Rehabilitation 18(1): 7–32.

Zimmerman TS, Prest LA, Wetzel BE (1997) Solution-focused couples therapy groups: an empirical study. Journal of Family Therapy 19: 125–44.

Index